COMMUNICATION IN PARKINSON'S DISEASE

Presented by

Roche Products Limited

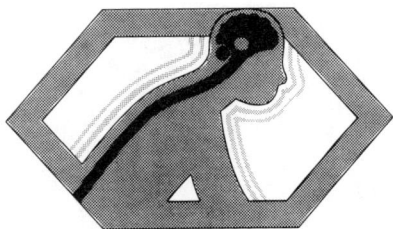

*Action in
Parkinson's Disease*

Roche Products Limited
PO Box 8, Welwyn Garden City
Hertfordshire AL7 3AY
Tel: Welwyn Garden 328128

COMMUNICATION IN PARKINSON'S DISEASE

SHEILA SCOTT, F.I. CAIRD and B.O. WILLIAMS

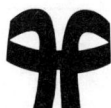

CROOM HELM
London & Sydney

© 1985 Sheila Scott, F.I. Caird and B.O. Williams
Croom Helm Ltd, Provident House, Burrell Row,
Beckenham, Kent BR3 1AT
Croom Helm Australia Pty Ltd, First Floor, 139 King Street,
Sydney, NSW 2001, Australia

British Library Cataloguing in Publication Data

Scott, Sheila, 1955-
 Communication in Parkinson's disease.
 1. Parkinsonism — Treatment 2. Speech
 therapy
 I. Title II. Caird, F.I. III. Williams, B.O.
 616.8'33   RC382

 ISBN 0-7099-2392-9

Typeset by Leaper & Gard Ltd, Bristol
Printed and bound in Great Britain
by Billing & Sons Limited, Worcester.

CONTENTS

FOREWORD

The striking advances of modern medicine are based on increasing understanding of normal physiology and its modification by disease. The treatment of Parkinson's disease was transformed by the recognition of dopaminergic neurones and of dopamine deficiency in the nigrostriatal pathways of the basal ganglia. An unfortunate corollary is a widespread tendency to overlook the possibilities of providing relief from symptoms which have unexplained mechanisms or of exploiting observations which cannot be explained by contemporary theory. Symptomatic relief of muscular rigidity by anticholinergic drugs and suppression of tremor by drugs or stereotaxic surgery still have a value, although their pathogenesis is not fully understood. In the nineteenth century it was recognised that many patients could be relieved by horse riding or by sitting on a vibrating chair, but the observation has not been exploited. When the abnormal mechanism is obscure or not amenable to correction, an operational approach is entirely respectable.

The authors of this book have not been daunted by the absence of an accepted basis for the disorders of speech and communication which are so common and distressing alike to patients and relatives. In the present state of knowledge an account of the pathology of Parkinsonism and the physiology and biochemistry of the basal ganglia would have little relevance. Their approach has been to analyse the dysprosody, dysphasia and articulatory problems of patients at a purely descriptive level and to devise rehabilitatory measures for these which are well within the scope of trained speech therapists. Their published results of preliminary work are sufficiently encouraging for this operational approach to justify further presentation of their methods and findings so that speech therapists and others responsible for the rehabilitation of patients with Parkinson's disease may use them.

J.A. Simpson,
Professor of Neurology,
University of Glasgow.

PREFACE

The limited information available about the nature and consequences of the speech disorder of Parkinson's disease provided the impetus for this text. Growing interest and increased study of this communication difficulty have substantiated the role of the speech therapist (or speech-language clinician) in the team approach to the disease. However, this increased interest has highlighted the insufficient literature available to therapists.

The aim of this text is to direct attention to the importance of speech therapy in the clinical management of such patients. The authors briefly review the nature of the disorder and the current medical management of the disease, and discuss in detail assessment guidelines and traditional and modern methods of speech therapy. We hope it will assist speech therapy students and therapists, and may prove of interest to other health professionals interested in Parkinson's disease.

The authors are grateful to Dr Ian Bone, Consultant Neurologist, Institute of Neurological Sciences, Glasgow, for his helpful advice and suggestions; to Dr Mike MacMahon, University of Glasgow, for his constructive criticism and interest; to Mrs Alison Beattie (Occupational Therapist) and Mr David McNiven (District Physiotherapist, South Eastern District, Glasgow) for their useful recommendations; to the Parkinson's Disease Society for their continuing support; and to Mrs Marisa Smith for her invaluable assistance with the manuscript.

1 THE NATURE AND NATURAL HISTORY OF PARKINSON'S DISEASE

Parkinson's disease, first described by Parkinson in 1817, is among the commoner neurological disorders; it affects older people in particular and makes a major impact on their lives and those of their relatives. Parkinsonism has a number of causes, but only the drug-induced form and that of unknown cause (so-called idiopathic Parkinson's disease) are numerically important. The form of Parkinsonism that followed epidemic encephalitis is now increasingly rare, as the sufferers from the last epidemic in the late 1920s and early 1930s progressively die.

The prevalence of Parkinson's disease has been studied in a number of continents and in a number of ways, but there is general agreement that its frequency increases almost exponentially with age (Figure 1.1; Broe *et al.*, 1976). It is rare under the age of 40 and becomes increasingly common thereafter. At any one time approximately half of the sufferers from the disease are over 70 years of age, and it is most commonly encountered in the seventh decade. A useful figure, and one easy to remember, is that at the age of 70 idiopathic Parkinson's disease affects approximately 1.5 per cent of all people, without definite distinction of sex.

Nevertheless, it must be remembered that although Parkinson's disease is a common condition, the average general practitioner will have no more than five patients with Parkinson's disease on his list at any one time, and he will perhaps see only one or two new patients each year. Considerations of management and of specialist advice must bear these facts in mind.

The prevalence of drug-induced Parkinsonism is not known, but it is certainly increasingly common in the elderly (Williamson, 1984). The common causes are the phenothiazine and butyrophenone groups of drugs (Table 1.1). Any elderly patient with newly discovered Parkinsonism requires a searching enquiry about current or previous drugs which may be implicated, since evident Parkinsonism may persist for as long as two years after the causal drug has been withdrawn. The majority of such patients however improve, the Parkinsonism regresses, and they require no specific treatment.

1

Figure 1.1: Age-specific Prevalence Rates of Parkinson's Disease:
▫—▫ Rochester (Minnesota) (Kurland, 1958); ○—○ Carlisle (UK)
(Brewis *et al.*, 1966); ●—● Victoria (Australia) (Jenkins, 1966); △—△
Iceland (Gudmundsson, 1966); ▲—▲ Baltimore (Maryland) (Kessler,
1972); ×—× Glasgow (UK) (Broe *et al.*, 1976)

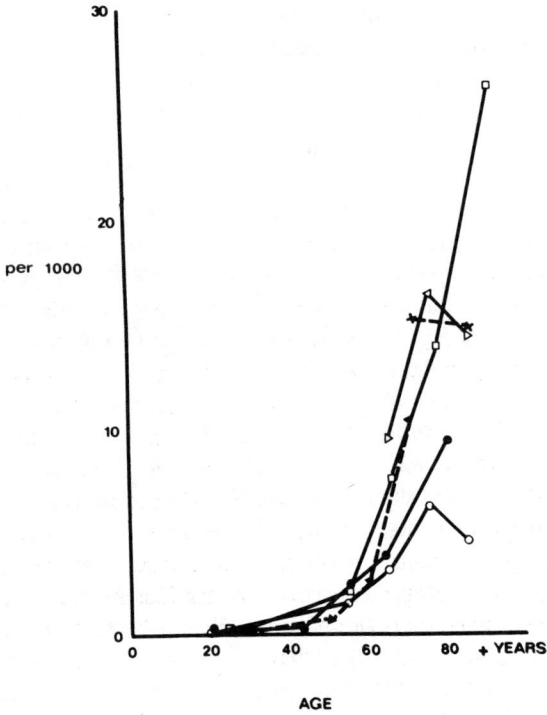

Source: Caird (1980).

Table 1.1: Drugs Which May Cause or Aggravate Parkinsonism

phenothiazines:	chlorpromazine
	promazine
	thioridazine
	prochlorperazine
butyrophenones:	haloperidol
	droperidol
methyldopa	
reserpine	

Pathology

The ultimate cause of Parkinson's disease seems to be a degeneration and loss of neurones in the dopaminergic systems in the substantia nigra and elsewhere in the brain, but other cell groups and systems there also appear to be involved, at least in patients who have had the condition for a decade or so. Together with this loss of neurones, there is a parallel decline in dopamine synthesis or in the enzymes responsible for it in the basal ganglia. The loss of nerve cells and of dopamine synthesis is of the order of 80 per cent of the young adult normal values in cases of mild Parkinson's disease, and 90-100 per cent in severe cases. The normal decline with age is approximately 50 per cent (itself a reduction greater than in most phsysiological functions) so that some additional factor is clearly at work, and the ageing process by itself is most unlikely to be the sole cause of Parkinson's disease. What the factor responsible is is quite unknown at present, but one clue is that cigarette smoking appears in part to protect against the disease.

Symptoms and Signs

The manifestations of Parkinson's disease are numerous and complex. The commonest, and those without which it cannot be diagnosed, are tremor, rest, rigidity of muscles, and bradykinesia, or slowness and poverty of movement.

The first symptom of which the patient complains is usually tremor of one hand, spreading after a variable period of months or years to affect the other hand and perhaps the legs and face.

Rigidity and poverty of movement are particularly important when the patient is in the horizontal position. Thus difficulty in turning in bed is one of the commonest disabilities of which patients complain. Difficulty in rising from a chair, in beginning to walk, in stopping walking (leading to the so-called festinating or hurrying gait), and impairment of balance, resulting in falls, may also be early features of the condition. Sufferers regularly say that they experience difficulty with fine finger movements, so that daily activities such as doing up buttons are frustrating. Micrographia is not uncommon (Figure 1.2).

Increased salivation, combined with difficulty in swallowing saliva, leading to drooling, and increased sebum secretion, which leads to a greasy skin, are also frequent.

The speech problems of the disease are described in detail later (Chapter 2), as is also the association between the various features of the condition and speech. In general the severity of the speech disorder is related to the severity of the disease, but there are notable exceptions to this rule.

When the patient is examined, the tremor is found to be, initially at least, regular and of moderate rapidity (4-6/sec). It affects particularly the thumb, thus producing the so-called pill-

Figure 1.2: Example of Micrographic Writing

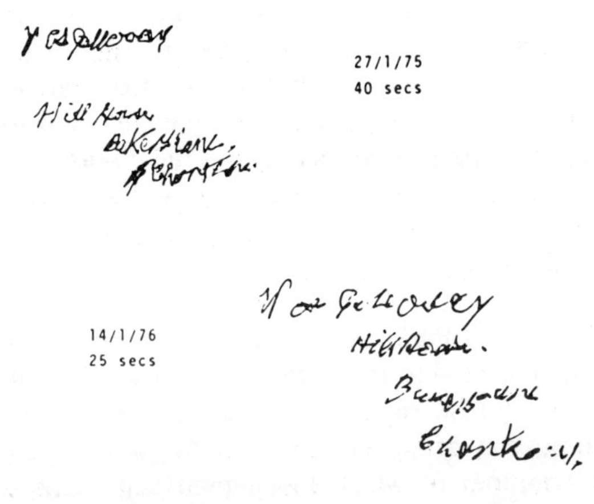
27/1/75
40 secs
14/1/76
25 secs

Source: Reproduced by kind permission of Roche Pharmaceuticals Ltd.

rolling phenomenon. The tremor is worse at rest and under stress, and it is abolished by movement, by sleep, and also interestingly by a stroke affecting the tremulous limb, as was noted by Parkinson himself.

Rigidity is seen in the upper limb as a plastic difficulty in flexing and extending the patient's wrist and elbow. It occurs similarly in the lower limbs at ankle, knee and hip; the neck muscles and those of the trunk are also affected. The combination of tremor and rigidity produces the so-called cog-wheel effect, best seen on flexion and extension of the wrist and/or elbow, over the biceps tendon. The impression is given of a cog-wheel or ratchet, as the tremor temporarily and repeatedly interrupts the rigidity.

Bradykinesia or poverty of movement is seen in the unblinking immobile mask-like face, the limited turning movements of the head, which combine to give the patient a curious tortoise-like appearance, and in slowness of initiation of movement. This is well seen when rapid alternating movements of the fingers are asked for, for instance as in mimicking piano-playing. Poverty of movement also particularly affects the so-called associated movements such as arm-swinging during walking. The body's responses to rapid displacement are reduced, and this is probably partly the reason for the falls to which Parkinsonian sufferers are especially prone. They have lost the normal speed of response to falling, and so cannot prevent this from happening.

The posture of the patient is characteristic, with the head, trunk, hips and knees slightly flexed (Figure 1.3). The gait is shuffling, with the feet appearing glued to the ground as the patient starts to walk. This can often be overcome by teaching him to twist the trunk to and fro, or to rock on to one foot, so that the opposite foot becomes as it were unglued.

The very common emotional and psychological consequences of the disease, in which problems with speech play a most important part, are discussed later (Chapter 4).

Natural History

The natural history of the untreated disease is now obscured by effective drug treatment but Parkinson's disease in general slowly progresses over a decade or more, with increasing disability and finally death usually from respiratory complications (Hoehn and

Figure 1.3: Characteristic Posture of Parkinson's Disease

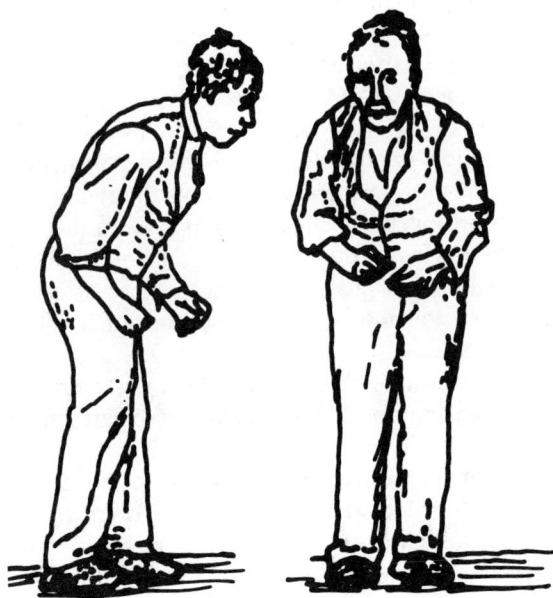

Paralysis agitans. (After St. Leger.)

Source: Reproduced by kind permission of Roche Pharmaceuticals Ltd.

Yahr, 1961). There are however a small number of patients in whom progression is much more rapid, so that they are severely disabled within a year or two of the onset, and at the other end of the spectrum another larger group (perhaps 10 per cent) in whom there appears to be no progression over the years and the condition remains stationary.

The treated condition shows a similar progress in many cases, and after ten years only one-third of patients remain free of major disability (Shaw *et al*, 1980; Pentland *et al.*, 1982). Treatment itself also has its own important complications (Williamson and Chopin, 1979; Hildick-Smith, 1980; see Chapter 6).

The most serious complication encountered in both the untreated and the treated natural history of the disease is the development of intellectual impairment. It does not respond to treatment, and occurs in a substantial proportion of patients (approximately 30 per cent), after 7-10 years or more of the disease. The present evidence suggests that this is part of the disease itself, in most cases at least, and *not* due to its treatment. Other common pathologies producing dementia, such as Alzheimer's disease, may also co-exist, particularly in elderly patients.

References

Brewis, M., Poskanzer, D.S., Rolland, C., Miller, H. (1966). Neurological disorders in an English city. *Acta Neurologica Scandinavica, 42* (Suppl. 24), 1-89.

Broe, G.A., Akhtar, A.J., Andrews, G.R., Caird, F.I., Gilmore, A.J.J., and MacLennan, W.J. (1976). Neurological disorders in the elderly. *Journal of Neurology, Neurosurgery and Psychiatry, 39*, 362-6.

Caird, F.I. (ed.) (1980). *Neurological Disorders in the Elderly.* Wright — PSG, Bristol.

Gudmusson, K.R. (1966). A clinical survey of Parkinsonism in Iceland. *Acta Neurologica Scandinavica, 43* (Suppl. 33), 1-61.

Hildick-Smith, M. (1980). Management of Parkinson's disease in the elderly. In M.J. Denham (ed.), *The Treatment of Medical Problems in the Elderly.* MTP Press, Lancaster, pp. 215-58.

Hoehn, M.M., and Yahr, M.D. (1967). Parkinsonism: onset, progression and mortality. *Neurology, 17* 427-42.

Jenkins, A.C. (1966). Epidemiology of Parkinsonism in Victoria. *Medical Journal of Australia, 2*, 496-502.

Kessler, I.I. (1972). Epidemiological studies of Parkinson's disease. Part 3: Community-based survey. *American Journal of Epidemiology, 96*, 242-54.

Kurland, L.T. (1958). Epidemiology, incidence, geographical distribution, and genetic considerations. In W.S. Fields (ed.),

Pathogenesis and Treatment of Parkinsonism. Charles C. Thomas, Springfield, Illinois, pp. 5-43.

Pentland, B., Matthews, D., and Maudsley, C. (1982). Parkinson's disease: long-term results of levodopa therapy. *Scottish Medical Journal, 27,* 284-7.

Shaw, K.M., Lees, A.J., and Stern, G.M. (1980). The impact of treatment with levodopa on Parkinson's disease. *Quarterly Journal of Medicine, NS49,* 283-93.

Williamson, J. (1984). Drug-induced Parkinson's disease. *British Medical Journal, 288,* 1457.

Williamson, J., and Chopin, J.M. (1979). Adverse reactions to prescribed drugs in the elderly: a multi-centre investigation. *Age and Ageing,* 73-80.

2 SPEECH SYMPTOMS IN PARKINSON'S DISEASE

In his original description of the disease, Parkinson gave only passing mention to some of the features characteristic of the speech disorder inherent in the condition. He noted in one subject in the later stages of the disease 'words are scarcely now intelligible'; in another case, he alluded to the 'impediment of speech' and said that speech was 'very much interrupted'. When referring to pathognomonic symptoms, he clearly recorded the difficulties encountered in posture, gait and walking, adding that 'a similar affection of the speech, when the tongue thus outruns the mind, is termed volubility'.

Modern accounts of Parkinson's disease include the changes in speech as an integral part of the disease process. Various descriptions of the speech manifestations are similar; one of the most comprehensive is that by Grewel (1957).

Articulation is slow and difficult. The voice is increasingly dysphonic, whilst speech is soft, blurred, irregular in rhythm and rate, and 'trailing' is noticed at the start. Thus the monotonous and slow speech of these patients gradually develops. They make an obvious use of short sentences, and sentence inflection is not only stereotyped, but its range is narrow and short. The other factors giving speech its expressiveness — loudness, rate and especially stress, inflection and intonation — are lost or reduced. The 'tune' of speech may disappear entirely in some cases. Consonants become blurred and elided, sometimes muffled. The voice, in the beginning breathy and hoarse, is increasingly dysphonic: it develops a nasal quality. Breathing disturbances interrupt phonation. Often slow speech accelerates during speaking.

Grewel also observed that a lack of speech propulsion was particularly characteristic of the disease in the advanced stages.

Incidence

Speech disorder is common in Parkinson's disease. Atarashi and Uchida (1959) claimed that the prevalence of dysarthric manifestations in Parkinsonism was as high as 73 per cent and Selby (1968) found disordered speech production in all of the cases he studied, although it is remarkable that almost half of all the subjects interviewed reported that their speech was unimpaired. (He found that gross speech difficulties were most common in post-encephalitic cases, rather than those presenting with idiopathic parkinsonism.) In a more recent study of 261 Parkinson's disease sufferers (Oxtoby, 1982), 49 per cent of those surveyed reported speech disturbances of a significant degree. Oxtoby commented that speech difficulties were responsible for some of the most embarrassing, upsetting and isolating aspects of Parkinson's disease.

It is thus generally accepted that speech disorder occurs in half of all cases: it becomes more prevalent as the disease progresses (Uziel *et al.*, 1975).

Classification

Traditionally the speech disorder has been classified as a dysarthria (Peacher, 1949) or more specifically as a dysarthrophonia, but this classification is unsatisfactory as the disorder is more complex. Lenneburg (1967) ascribed the speech manifestations to an 'adisdochokinesia of voice', the dysarthria being merely concomitant of a condition that affects the whole facial and oral musculature. All the features are generally attributed to hypokinesia, considered a cardinal feature of the disease (Mawdsley and Gamsu, 1971).

Darley *et al.* (1975) defined clusters of deviant speech dimensions that are characteristic of various types of dysarthria, based upon the underlying disturbed neurophysiology. The analysis of the dysarthria of Parkinson's disease led to the redefinition of this speech disorder in terms of respiration, phonation, articulation and prosody. They have provided therapists with the most comprehensive method of identification of dysarthria since the holistic approach of Peacher (1949).

In their perceptual studies Darley *et al.* (1969a, b) reported that the most prominent features of hypokinetic dysarthria are:

(1) A monotony of pitch, reduced stress, and a monotony of loudness.

(2) An imprecision of articulation, resulting in a 'blur of speech'.
(3) Speech is often arrested, resulting in inappropriate silences and sometimes repetitions of phonemes and syllables.
(4) Speech is produced in short rushes. The rate is often variable.
(5) Vocal quality is often breathy.

Scott and Caird (1981) have suggested that the speech disorder of Parkinson's disease is more appropriately considered as a dysprosody.

Respiration

Much controversy remains about the effects of the disease on respiratory function. Darley *et al.* (1975) suggested that there is limited excursion of the respiratory and phonatory muscles like other muscles. Objective assessments of respiration have revealed irregular and inflexible breathing patterns, poor synchronisation of respiration with speech, and a marked reduction in vital capacity. De la Torre *et al.* (1960) noted reduced vital capacity and more significantly irregular breathing cycles. They attributed this to disruption of the normal agonist-antagonist synergy in the respiratory muscles. Laszewski (1956) attributed the reduction in vital capacity to the rigidity of the articulatory musculature rather than a restriction of the respiratory muscles. Kim (1968) considered that the rigidity of the chest musculature and the resultant limited amplitude of respiration might in part explain the reduction and variability in vocal intensity present in Parkinsonian speech. Mueller (1971) substantiated this, finding that his control group expired significantly larger volumes of air during sustained phonation on /a/ than sufferers from Parkinson's disease. An interesting influence on respiratory function was reported by Ewanowski (1964). Under controlled conditions verbal reinforcement caused Parkinsonian subjects to perform as well as controls during sustained phonation on isolated vowels.

? possible effect of singing on respiration function

Phonation

Darley *et al.* (1975) considered that the salient feature of hypo-kinesia manifests itself particularly in the phonatory aspects of speech.

Studies by Canter (1963a, b) and Kammermeier (1969) suggested that male Parkinsonian speakers exhibit higher than normal vocal pitch levels. The pitch levels displayed are more characteristic of an older age group of apparently normal men.

Parkinsonian speakers are generally considered to have reduced pitch variability, using a range of pitch levels more restricted than those used by normal subjects and their speech is considered to display less speech inflection; this was recorded as long ago as 1925 by Schilling.

Vocal Quality

Lehiste (1965) studied the acoustic patterns of a Parkinsonian subject and concluded that the efficiency of phonation in Parkinson's disease is reduced. Sufferers are considered to have difficulty synchronising phonation and respiration. Cisler (1927) noted that closure of the glottis was limited in Parkinson's disease and that vocal cord movement did not synchronise with articulatory movement, resulting in a breathy or hoarse vocal quality.

Vocal Intensity

Canter (1963) studied the vocal intensity levels of male Parkinsonian speakers and matched normals. He noted that the two groups did not vary in mean peak sound pressure levels, but the normal subjects were able to produce a larger range of vocal intensity levels in speech, their control over these being considerably better. Parkinsonian subjects were unable to achieve the delicate control of subglottic pressure necessary for quiet phonation, and they could not match the level of loud phonation achieved by the control group.

Prosodic Studies

It seems strange that although both Monrad-Krohn (1947) and Darley *et al.* (1975) considered the salient features of the speech disorder as affecting the prosody of speech, so much emphasis has been placed upon the purely dysarthric aspects. Prosody may be defined as the patterned distribution of stress, intonation and other phonatory features in speech. In effective communication, the prosodic and suprasegmental features of intonation, tone of voice, and stress contribute greatly to the determination of the implied meaning and to the overall intelligibility of the speaker. Misuse of pause and rhythm, and distortion of intonation can severely impair speech intelligibility despite competent articulation.

Stress is commonly perceived as an increase in intensity of a syllable in conjunction with altered syllable length. In English improper use of stress severely affects intelligibility. Stress may also be contrastive, permitting noun-verb distinctions (see Appendix 5):

e.g. récord vs. recórd

Stress also permits similar words which are spelled the same way or sound the same, but are unrelated in meaning, to be distinguished by ear:

e.g. désert (a sandy place)   dèsert (to run away)

Intonation contributes to the overall meaning of words and sentences. It is considered by many linguists to be a primary aspect of language development, and possibly this is the reason that it is so resistant to change or to therapeutic intervention. Intonation also enables us to convey different emotions at a single word level, e.g., 'yes' may be definite, eager or doubtful.

Scott and Caird (1983) recently emphasised the importance of prosodic impairment of speech in Parkinson's disease and its influence upon intelligibility. It is generally accepted that imprecise articulation is a feature of the speech of Parkinson's disease (Canter, 1965b), but Scott and Caird could find only one in a sample of 55 Parkinsonian subjects who made articulatory errors. All the others examined appeared to have articulatory deviances, but phonological analysis carried out by two therapists independently did not confirm this impression. Dysprosody mimicked disordered articulation. Certainly reduction in the abnormal prosodic features by therapy improved the impression of articulatory impairment and general unintelligibility, a phenomenon supported by Rosenbek and La Pointe (1978).

Rate

The speaking rate of Parkinsonian sufferers appears to be faster than that of normal speakers. Analysis has revealed that rate is particularly increased in segments of contextual speech and that speech tends to be produced in short rushes. Studies of oral reading rates have revealed a wide range of words per minute (Kreul, 1972; Kammermeier, 1969) and it is generally accepted that although Parkinsonian patients do not appear to be statistically different from normal control groups, there is considerable individual variation and that there are some Parkinsonian subjects for whom reduced or accelerated reading and speaking rates represent a major feature of their speech disturbance (Canter, 1965a, b).

Oral diadochokinetic studies have produced varying results. Sufferers from Parkinson's disease tend to have great difficulty producing rapid repetitions of phonemes discretely. They display a slowness of rate and dysrhythmia, and have difficulty maintaining vocal intensity throughout the exercise (Kreul, 1972).

Resonance

Nasal resonance is often considered to be impaired in the speech of Parkinson's disease (Mueller, 1971), but Cisler (1927) found no measurable nasal airflow during speech in the subjects studied. Darley *et al.* (1975) agreed that speech might sound hypernasal, but analysis revealed that this was not significant and that no nasal emission of air was found.

Drug Effects

The effects of drug treatment upon the speech of Parkinson's disease are discussed in Chapter 6, but the overall intelligibility of speech can remain distorted despite otherwise optimal drug therapy (Scott and Caird, 1981).

Receptive Disorder

Parkinson's disease is usually considered to be a pure disorder of
movement, but there is some evidence of subtle receptive disorders, involving especially visual and spatial perception (Villardita *et
al.*, 1966). A recent study (Scott *et al.*, 1984) has suggested that there
is also an element of perceptual difficulty present in the speech difficulties of the disease. During a trial to determine the possible benefits
of speech therapy for Parkinson's disease sufferers, it became apparent that they were unable to appreciate the prosodic features of intonation and stress in their own speech production or in the speech of
others. They also appeared to have difficulty in appreciating different
patterns of facial expression, failing to note the additional clues to
speech presented by facial gesture.

Parkinsonian subjects and matched apparently normal elderly
counterparts were assessed on seven tests of prosodic appreciation:
discrimination of prosodic contrasts, matching cartoon pictures of
facial expression to contextual speech clues (Figure 2.1), discrimination of the affective and grammatical functions of prosody,

Figure 2.1: Cartoon Facial Expressions

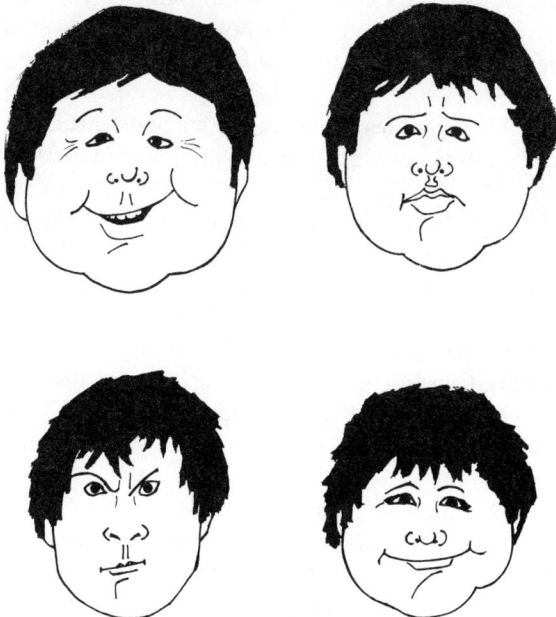

discrimination of the semantic function of prosody, and on three tests of expression (production of a neutral statement, angry tones, and questioning tones). There was a significant difference between the two groups in all the tests except those of prosodic contrast and in the production of a neutral statement. The greatest difference was in the ability to evaluate facial expression and intonation. These receptive difficulties in addition to the obvious motor problems may have important clinical and therapeutic implications.

References

Atarashi, J., and Uchida, E. (1959). A clinical study of Parkinsonism. *Recent Advances in Research in the Nervous System, 3*, 871-82.

Canter, G.J. (1963). Speech characteristics of patients with Parkinson's disease. I. Intensity, pitch and duration. *Journal of Speech and Hearing Disorders, 28*, 221-9.

_____ (1965a). Speech characteristics of patients with Parkinson's disease. II. Physiological support for speech. *Journal of Speech and Hearing Disorders, 30*, 44-9.

_____ (1965b). Speech characteristics of patients with Parkinson's disease. III. Articulation diadochokinesis, and overall speech adequacy. *Journal of Speech and Hearing Disorders, 30*, 217-24.

Cisler, I. (1927). Sur les troubles du language articulé et de la phonation au cours de l'encéphalite epidémique. *Arch. Int. Laryngol., 6*, 1054-7.

Cramer, W. (1940). De spraak bij patienten met Parkinsonisme. *Logopedie en Foniatrie, 22*, 17-23.

Darley, F.L., Aronson, A.E., and Brown, J.R. (1969a). Differential diagnostic patterns of dysarthria. *Journal of Speech and Hearing Research, 12*, 246-69.

_____ (1969b). Clusters of deviant speech dimensions in the dysarthrias. *Journal of Speech and Hearing Research, 12*, 462-96.

_____ (1975). *Motor Speech Disorders.* W.B. Saunders Co., Philadelphia, pp. 171-93.

De la Torre, R., Mier, M., and Boshes, B. (1960). Studies in Parkinsonism. IX. Evaluation of respiratory function: preliminary observations. *Quarterly Bulletin Northwest University Medical School, 34*, 332-6.

Ewanowski, S.J. (1964). Selected motor-speech behaviour of patients with Parkinsonism. PhD dissertation, University of Wisconsin.

Grewel, F. (1957). Dysarthria in post-encephalitic Parkinsonism. *Acta Psychiatrica neurologica Scandinavica, 32,* 444-7.

Kammermeier, M.A. (1969). A comparison of phonatory phenomena among groups of neurologically impaired speakers. PhD dissertation, University of Minnesota.

Kim, R. (1968). The chronic residual respiratory disorder in post-encephalitic Parkinsonism. *Journal of Neurology, Neurosurgery and Psychiatry, 31,* 393-8.

Kreul, E.J. (1972). Neuromuscular control examination (NMC) for Parkinsonism: vowel prolongations and diadochokinet and reading rates. *Journal of Speech and Hearing Research, 15,* 72-83.

Laszewski, Z. (1956). Role of the department of rehabilitation in preoperative evaluation of Parkinsonian patients. *Journal of the American Geriatrics Society, 4,* 1280-4.

Leanderson, R., Meyerson, B.A., and Persson, A. (1971). Effect of L-dopa on speech in Parkinsonism. *Journal of Neurology, Neurosurgery and Psychiatry, 34,* 679-81.

Lehiste, I. (1965). Some acoustic characteristics of dysarthric speech. *Bibliothea Phonetica,* Fasc. 2. Basel: S. Karger.

Lenneberg, E.H. (1967). *The Biological Foundations of Language.* Wiley, New York.

Mawdsley, C., and Gamsu, C.V. (1971). Periodicity of speech in Parkinsonism. *Nature, 231,* 315-6.

Monrad-Krohn, G.H. (1947). Dysprosody or altered melody of language. *Brain, 70 (iv),* 405.

Mueller, P.B. (1971). Parkinson's disease. Motor speech behaviour in a selected group of patients. *Folia Phoniatrica, 23,* 333-46.

Mysak, E.D. (1959). Pitch and duration characteristics of older males. *Journal of Speech and Hearing Research, 2,* 46-54.

Oxtoby, M. (1982). *Parkinson's Disease Patients and their Social Needs.* Parkinson's Disease Society, London.

Peacher, W.G. (1949). Aetiology and differential diagnosis of dysarthria. *Journal of Speech and Hearing Disorders, 15,* 252-65.

Rosenbek, J.C., and La Pointe, L.L. (1978). The dysarthrias: description, diagnosis and treatment. In F.D. Johns (ed.), *Clinical Management of Neurogenic Communicative Disorders,*

Little, Brown & Co., Boston, pp. 251-310.

Scott, S., and Caird, F.I. (1981). Speech therapy for patients with Parkinson's disease. *British Medical Journal, 283*, 1088.

_____ (1983). Speech therapy for Parkinson's disease. *Journal of Neurology, Neurosurgery and Psychiatry, 46*, 140-4.

Scott, S., Caird, F.I., and Williams, B.O. (1984). Evidence for an apparent sensory speech disorder in Parkinson's disease. *Journal of Neurology, Neurosurgery and Psychiatry* (in press).

Schilling, R. (1925). Experimentalphonetische Untersuchungen bei Erhrankungen des Extrapyramidalen Systems. *Archiv für Psychiatrie und Nervenkrankheiten, 75*, 419-71.

Selby, G. (1968). Parkinson's disease. In P.J. Vinken and G.W. Bruyn (eds.), *Handbook of Clinical Neurology, Vol 6*. North Holland Publishing Company, Amsterdam.

Uziel, A., Bohe, M., Cadilhac, J., and Passouant, P. (1975). Les troubles de la voix et de la parole dans les syndromes Parkinsoniens. *Folia Phoniatrica, 27*, 166-76.

Villardita, C., Smirni, P., Le Pira, F., Zappala, G., and Nicoletti, F. (1966). Mental deterioration, visuoperceptive disabilities and constructional apraxia in Parkinson's Disease. *Acta Neurologica Scandinavica, 1*, 114-120.

3 NON-PARKINSONIAN INFLUENCES ON SPEECH IN PARKINSON'S DISEASE

Assessment in dysarthria is designed to establish what symptoms are present and to measure their severity, to define the speech diagnosis, and as far as possible rationalise speech therapy. This necessitates recording the presence of co-existing disorders, or excluding ruling them out, since they might influence the outcome of therapy or the patient's ability to co-operate. It is important that the therapist does not forget these other influences upon speech deterioration (Wertz, in Johns, 1978).

Ageing

Any discussion of the communication impairment characteristic of Parkinson's disease must be considered within the general framework of the ageing process. It is accepted that with age, people experience physical, psychological and cognitive changes, although the view taken today is fortunately not as pessimistic as that of Aristotle, who believed that man advanced up to the age of 50 years and after that time, physical decline of the body carried the whole person downhill.

Undoubtedly changes in a variety of modalities of sensation and in perception associated with ageing have considerable influence upon the performance of the elderly. They occur alongside and together with those of neurological disease.

Vision

Efficient vision plays an important role in the individual's ability to respond to his environment, including those who are trying to communicate with him. Without accurate vision it is impossible to interpret the non-verbal clues of facial expression, listener/speaker distance and more specifically lip movements, which are all vital in effective communication (Greene, 1982).

The reasons for visual deterioration in old age are varied: they include retinal disease, loss of lens elasticity or clarity, and cloud-

19

ing of the cornea. Senile cataract, glaucoma, macular degeneration and ocular disease secondary to long-standing systemic conditions are almost universal in old age (Freeman, 1960). Botwinick (1973) suggests that by the age of 70, without correction, poor vision is the rule rather than the exception. As with other disabilities elderly people tend not to report visual problems, accepting their difficulties as an inevitable part of ageing.

No specific ocular abnormalities occur in Parkinson's disease, although, particularly in post-encephalitic cases, many eye signs exist. These include blepharospasm, blepharoclonus and (only in post-encephalitic cases) oculogyric crises.

Hearing

Hearing loss may have devastating effects upon communication. The individual with slowly deteriorating hearing is faced with the prospect of gradual estrangement from associates and family (Yarrington, 1976). Hearing deteriorates with age, and has been described as the greatest barrier to social interaction and personal adjustment (Hinchcliffe, 1983). Presbyacusis can account for difficulties not only in hearing the high tones of speech, but also in its comprehension. It may lead to irritation and unhappiness. Relationships with the decreasing numbers of people close to the old person can become extremely strained.

Presbyacusis involves all of the major divisions of both the peripheral and central auditory mechanisms, affecting frequency discrimination, temporal integration and loudness increment. Hearing aids therefore have to be considered as communication improvers. With proper prescription, advice and follow-up, modern hearing aids are essential to the preservation of reasonable communication skills (Bamford, 1983).

Motor Speech Function

Enderby (1980) pointed out that there is limited knowledge of the effects of ageing upon the motor speech skills. The features of speech impairment typical in Parkinson's disease (e.g. phonation, respiration and prosody) may well undergo changes with age. These may well be important to the recognition and assessment of communication problems. Greene (1980) has indicated that the physiological changes in the anatomical structures with age must adversely influence the force, rate and manner of muscular movement.

Respiration

Elderly people are much more susceptible to respiratory disease, particularly if they have been smokers (Addington and Agarwal, 1974). The effects of decreased lung tissue elasticity, reduced vital capacity and structural changes in the muscles of the thoracic cage result in reduced lung function (Kahane, 1981; Anderson and Williams, 1983), but these changes appear to have no demonstrable effects on the voice or other aspects of communication (Meyerson, 1976). Certainly the maximum values of respiratory volume necessary to sustain intra-oral air pressure and vowel duration greatly exceed the requirements for speech production. The vital capacity function is known to decrease proportionately with age. However, the ageing person can sustain a fair reduction in vital capacity before speech will be observed to suffer (Schow *et al.*, 1978). Vital capacity (the maximum volume of air which is expired after the maximum inspiration) is responsible for the control of vocal volume, maintaining pitch, intonation and voice resonance.

Canter (1963, 1965) studied duration of phonation and respiratory volumes and recorded no significant difference in volume or duration between the subjects with Parkinsonism and the age and sex matched normals.

Ryan (1972) noted a slight increase in vocal intensity with ageing after the age of 70 years. Ryan and Burke (1974) considered that the listener often judged a speaker's age from his voice. They suggested that laryngeal air loss, laryngeal tension, voice tremor, imprecise consonants, and slow articulation were reliable predictors of a speaker's age, and that these features of speech should form the basis of therapy in the vocal rehabilitation of the elderly.

Laryngeal Function

Anatomical and physiological changes with age include ossification of cartilages of the larynx, atrophy of the muscles of the vocal folds (which is responsible for the elevated fundamental frequency of ageing males — Mysack, 1959), stiffening of the crico-arytenoid joints and perhaps declining endocrine function as it affects the larynx (Luchsinger and Arnold, 1965).

Resonance

There are few reports concerning age changes in nasal resonance in speech. Hutchinson *et al.* (1978) examined velopharyngeal function and found that changes in the velopharyngeal mechanism occuring with age resulted in mild velopharyngeal incompetence. Changes in the thoracic skeleton with age may also contribute to change in resonance. In a similar way neuro-muscular deterioration, ill-fitting dentures and hearing loss may all affect speech resonance.

Articulation

Rate of speaking is known to decline steadily with age. Ptacek *et al.* (1966) described reduced diadochokinetic rates for lip and tongue movements in subjects over 65 years of age. Generally these changes in function have been attributed to the effects of ageing upon the neuromusculature, but Hutchinson and Beasley (1976) have suggested that the imprecision might be the result of inadequate sensory proprioception.

Many elderly speakers are considered to have slurred speech and Ryan and Burke (1974) have postulated that the older speakers might lie at the mild end of the continuum of dysarthria. The everyday occurrence of ill-fitting dentures (an easily remedied condition) may also influence articulatory accuracy and rate, marring otherwise good speech.

Prosody

Little is recorded about prosodic changes in the 'normal' elderly. Daniloff and Hammerberg (1973) have inferred that the demonstrable effects of age upon the articulatory mechanism may alter the prosody of speech. While in the opinion of Manning and Shirkey (1981), increased fluency breaks are seen in normal ageing, they may be explained by articulatory change such as slow rate, overall decrease in neuromuscular efficiency and imprecise articulation. In our own experience the ablity to perceive subtle functions of prosody used in expressing sarcasm, elliptical speech and abstract humour diminishes with age. Speech hesitation and repetition are recognised features of conversation in the elderly.

Dementia

Parkinson reported that the senses and intellect were uninjured in Parkinson's disease. A resumé of recent literature on intellectual functioning of patients with Parkinson's disease (Fisher and

Findley, 1981) has suggested that there is still controversy; there is an association between the disease and degrees of dementia.

Determining the presence of dementia is difficult, since one has to separate gross motor retardation, advancing age and mood changes from the effects of drug toxicity. There is little doubt that dementia is a feature of advanced Parkinson's disease, but may result from drug influences, rather than from the disease itself.

Matthews and Haaland (1979) reinforced the work of Monrad–Krohn (1947), who considered that the impoverished facial expression of Parkinson's disease belied the level of intellectual acuity and led to a false impression of apathy, depression and loss of intellect. They commented that the application of the term dementia to these patients is often grossly misleading and inaccurate.

The problem remains that accurate diagnosis and management of intellectual failure in these subjects is complicated by the lack of normal values for appropriate tests, and material uninfluenced by the effects of age and gross motor disturbance.

Dysphasia

It is not usually difficult to differentiate the dysarthria of Parkinson's disease from the language disorders of dysphasia. However, patients with Parkinson's disease who have suffered bilateral strokes or who have undergone unsuccessful bilateral thalamotomy are sometimes impossible to classify. In cases with more severely affected speech, the reduced verbal flow and general immobility may make assessment almost impossible.

Drug Side-effects

See Chapter 7.

References

Addington, W.W., and Agarwal, M.K. (1974). Managing reversible complications of chronic obstructive pulmonary disease in ambulatory patients. *Geriatrics, 29,* 76-83.

Anderson, W.F. and Williams, B.O. (eds) (1983). *Practical Management of the Elderly.* Blackwell, Oxford.

Bamford, J. (1983). Hearing and ageing. In Edwards, M. (ed.), *Communication Changes in Elderly People.* College of Speech Therapists, London.

Botwinick, J. (1973). *Ageing and Behaviour.* Springer, New York, p. 121.

Canter, G.J. (1963). Speech characteristics of patients with Parkinson's disease. I. Intensity, pitch and duration. *Journal of Speech and Hearing Disorders, 28,* 221-9.

_____ (1965). Speech characteristics of patients with Parkinson's disease. II. Physiological support for speech. *Journal of Speech and Hearing Disorders, 30,* 44-9.

Daniloff, R.G., and Hammerberg, R.F. (1973). In defining co-articulation. *Journal of Phonetics, 1,* 239

Enderby, P. (1980). Frenchay Dysarthria Assessment. *British Journal of Disorders of Communication, 15,* 165.

Fisher, K., and Findley, L. (1981). Intellectual changes in optimally treated patients with Parkinson's Disease. In Rose, F.C., and Capildeo, R. (eds), *Research Progress in Parkinson's Disease, II.* Pitman Medical, London, pp. 53-9.

Freeman, J. (1960). The geriatric limb on the gerontology tree. In Shock, N.W. (ed.), *Ageing: Some Social and Biological Aspects.* American Association for the Advancement of Science, Chicago.

Gardner, W.G. (1975). Hearing loss: the route to senility. *Audecibel, 24,* 74-6.

Greene, M.C.L. (1980). *The Voice and its Disorders,* 3rd edn. Pitman Medical, London.

_____ (1982). Ageing and the voice. In Edwards, M. (ed.), *Communication Changes in Elderly People.* College of Speech Therapists, London, pp. 62-7.

Hinchcliffe, R. (ed.) (1983). *Hearing and Balance in the Elderly.* Churchill Livingstone, London.

Hutchinson, J.M., Robinson, K.L., and Nerbonne, M.A. (1978). Patterns of nasalance in a sample of normal gerontologic subjects. *Journal of Communication Disorders, 11,* 469.

Johns, D.F. (ed.) (1978). *Clinical Management of Neurogenic Communication Disorders.* Little, Brown & Co., Boston, pp. 86-7.

Kahane, J.C. (1981). Changes in ageing: peripheral speech

mechanisms. In Beasley, D.S., and Davis, G.A. (eds), *Ageing Communication Processes and Disorders.* Grune & Stratton, New York.

Luchsinger, R., and Arnold, G.T. (1965). *Voice-Speech-Language.* Wadsworth, Belmont, California.

Manning, W.H., and Shirkey, E.A. (1981). Fluency and the ageing process. In Beasley, D.S., and Davis, G.A. (eds), *Aging: Communication Processes and Disorders.* Grune & Stratton, New York.

Matthews, C.G., and Haaland, K.Y. (1979). The effect of symptom deviation on cognitive and motor performance in Parkinsonism. *Neurology, 29,* 951-6.

Meyerson, M. (1976). The effects of ageing on communication. *Journal of Gerontology, 31,* 29-38.

Monrad-Krohn, G.H. (1947). Dysprosody or altered melody of language. *Brain, 70,* 405-8.

Mueller, P.B. (1971). Parkinson's Disease. Motor speech behaviour in a selected group of patients. *Folia Phoniatrica, 23,* 333-46.

Mysack, E.D. (1959). Pitch and duration characteristics of older males. *Journal of Speech and Hearing Research, 2,* 46-54.

Ptacek, P.H., Sonder, E.K., Maloney, W.H., and Jackson, C. (1966). Phonatory and related changes with advanced age. *Journal of Speech and Hearing Research, 9,* 353-60.

Ryan, W.J. (1972). Acoustic aspects of the ageing voice. *Journal of Gerontology, 27,* 265-7.

Ryan, W.J., and Burke, K.W. (1974). Perceptual and acoustic correlates of ageing in the speech of males. *Journal of Communication Disorders, 7,* 181.

Schow, R.L., Christenson, J.M., Hutchinson, J.M., and Nerbonne, M.A. (eds) (1978). *Communication Disorders of the Aged.* University Park Press, Baltimore.

Yarrington, C.T. Jr. (1976). Presbycusis. In Northern, J. (ed.), *Hearing Disorders.* Little, Brown & Co., Boston.

4 SOCIAL CONSEQUENCES OF THE COMMUNICATION DISORDER

In the first century B.C. Cicero wrote an essay 'De Senectute' (On Old Age), in which he regarded ageing as a normal aspect of life and he suggested that it is not old age which is at fault but our attitude to it. This view might also describe the problems inherent in Parkinson's disease: our attitude to the sufferer does much to influence his social isolation. Le Fevre (1959) stressed that the need to communicate does not lessen with an increase in physical disability. On the contrary the ability to communicate becomes more important in maintaining a level of social involvement. Impairment in communication interferes with the fundamental processes of social adjustment (Bloomer, 1955).

Certainly the effects of communication impairment can be devastating. The sufferer is no longer in control of his environment, is more dependent, and becomes embarrassed and withdrawn from social involvement, all of which lead to social isolation. Increasing difficulty in expressing emotions leads to frustration and despondency. The ability to impart information diminishes, and medical measures are thus limited because the sufferer cannot convey a full understanding of his problems.

Parkinson's disease does not kill immediately, but it can be a crippling condition with a strong tendency for increasing disability as time passes. Parkes (1982) considered that the patient should be encouraged to stay at work for as long as possible; it may be many years before normal activities are compromised.

The patient and his family need to know the prognosis of Parkinsonism. Both need reassurance that the illness is not psychological in origin nor due to stress, accidents, neglect, brain tumours or alcohol abuse, and that it is not contagious. Parkes (1982) has stressed that relatives should be advised that the patient cannot 'pull himself together'; rather, he requires positive, sympathetic encouragement.

In a survey of the social sequelae of the costs of Parkinsonism in 1972, Singer noted a reduction in daily activity, decreased income, and lessened ability in household management. There was an increased reliance on purely passive leisure activities, such as

26

watching television, and a marked reduction in the number of close friendships enjoyed by the sufferer. All of these are factors leading to social isolation, itself an important causal factor in depression, and to reduced interpersonal communication. Butfield (1961) stressed the importance of keeping alive a desire to communicate, emphasising the importance of a communicating environment. If people are not given the opportunity to communicate, they lose the will to talk.

Corollary in the opposite

The Social Consequences of Speech Difficulties

In the past, the attitudes of speech therapists have done little to relieve these difficulties which are encountered by both relatives and sufferers. They believed that little could be done to help or to alter the condition beyond the improvement brought about by drugs, and this resulted in non-referral to and non-intervention by speech therapists. There was all too often passive acceptance of this situation by sufferers and relatives alike.

Fortunately these attitudes are changing. Therapists are now involving themselves in the care of Parkinsonian patients, counselling relatives and communicating the need for intervention to other health care professionals.

The aim of management in the communication disorder of Parkinson's disease is to enable the patient to retain independence and maximise the use of residual communicating skills. As one might expect, sufferers are very distressed by their inability to speak with their accustomed ease and clarity. Dalton and Hardcastle (1977) highlighted that such radical changes in the sufferer's personal vocal image may lead to misunderstanding. Listeners believe that there has been a change of personality in the sufferer, or become frustrated by being unable to hear the inaudible flow of speech. Misunderstanding and requests for repetition increase the sufferer's anxiety and his inability to communicate effectively, and so create yet more frustration and tension.

Many mistake the sufferer's rapid mumblings for the wanderings of loss of intellect. The mumbled speech in conjunction with difficulties of balance and posture often lead to an impression of drunkeness, particularly in men, much to the embarrassment and distress of the sufferer.

The therapist must be aware of such problems, and not only

concentrate on advice on the physical speech and swallowing problems, but equally must help the family and sufferer adjust to and accept the changes in behaviour and attitude.

During a trial to evaluate the efficacy of speech therapy for Parkinson's disease Scott and Caird (1983) required relatives to comment on the speech changes in the subjects, before and after therapy, to estimate the degree of social difficulties encountered as a result of communication problems and their effects upon independent living. These difficulties are detailed in Table 4.1.

Most of the problems result in a need for increased supervision on the part of a relative. Following intensive therapy, improvement was noted in all of the items mentioned. Indeed it was commented upon in respect of several patients in whom relatives had initially recognised no problem. This highlighted the relatives' acceptance 'that it was all part of the illness and cannot be helped'.

Table 4.1: Difficulties of Communication Described by Relatives of Parkinsonian Sufferers before Speech Therapy

1. Problems with volume of the voice of the sufferer.
2. Difficulty in maintaining conversation because of monotonous responses.
3. Distress at the quality of the voice.
4. Difficulty in following the disordered rate of speech.
5. Embarrassment at their own inability to cope.
6. Difficulties for the sufferer using the telephone.

Social Consequences of Feeding Difficulties

The drooling, swallowing and eating problems of many sufferers often cause considerable embarrassment. Many families withdraw from social activities to avoid revealing this. Eating becomes a trial. Tremor or rigidity influence the use of and the control over cutlery. The occupational therapy aids described in Chapter 9 may help with these difficulties. Sufferers often complain about their spouses over-protecting or 'mothering' them, which they find demoralising. Frequently the family takes to having separate meal times from the sufferer, increasing his social isolation. Parkes (1982) considered problems of swallowing and chewing uncommon; however, Oxtoby (1982) reported that over 40 per cent of her sample complained of drooling and 26 per cent of swallowing difficulties. These difficulties and difficulty in retaining dentures and excessive salivation result in unsightly and messy table habits.

Social Sequelae

Physical and communication difficulties cause loss of confidence, and immobility. Sufferers resign from social and club activities. Many cease to attend church; this can be particularly distressing to previously regular attenders, and highlights their loss of belonging. Organised religion provides a social centre and a caring community. It is often a life-line for the housebound, especially through telephone communication, which is itself a medium inappropriate to those with disordered communication.

Loss of effective communication skills results in dependence upon third parties, such as doctors, visitors and others, to translate or to interpret their needs. Sufferers regret their loss of privacy and independence and may convey an incorrect impression both with their voice and face and this may be further misinterpreted by others. Despite such serious disease effects, only a minority of patients are unable to benefit from active involvement in the world around them. In Parkinsonism it is certain that much of the mental distress suffered by patients could be reduced by improved social awareness in others.

Parkinson's Disease Society

In the United Kingdom the Parkinson's Disease Society has been developed to aid sufferers of the disease and their relatives. It is a voluntary body active both in raising funds for research and in aiding the welfare of patients.

The local branches, of which the Society is in reality a part, are also of great value. They raise money for research into the disease and for numerous practical aspects of assistance for sufferers and caring relatives. They convey knowledge about the disease to sufferers, relatives and the general public and about how they themselves can help to combat its effects. In recent years it has been shown that local branches can greatly assist by directly employing the assistance of occupational, physiotherapists and speech therapists on a part-time basis, in this process of teaching of patients and their relatives. Practical guidance and help with particular problems can also be given to individual sufferers in the same way. It may well be that similar systems will be developed to a greater extent in the future.

In recent years the Society has been conducting a number of unique experiments such as 'therapeutic holidays', which combine treatment and welfare for the sufferers during such periods, thus relieving their carers.

Other comparable societies exist on the continent of Europe, in the United States and in Australasia, but they do not have the national appeal that the United Kingdom Society has. A list of useful local contact addresses is available from the Parkinson's Disease Society and some are given in Appendix 1.

References

Bloomer, H.H. (1955). Defective speech: a source of breakdown in communication. In Edwards, M. (ed.) (1982), *Communication Changes in Elderly People*. College of Speech Therapists, London.

Butfield, E. (1961). Dysarthria. *Speech Pathology and Therapy, 4,* 74.

Cicero, B.C. (106-43 b.c.). *De Senectute* (On Old Age). Translated by Copley, F. (1967) University of Michigan Press, Ann Arbor.

Dalton, P., and Hardcastle, W.J. (1977). *Disorders of Fluency: Studies in Language Disability and Remediation Series, No. 3.* Edward Arnold, London.

Le Fevre, M. (1959). Speech therapy for the geriatric patient. *Geriatrics, 12,* 691-5.

Oxtoby, M. (1982). *Parkinson's Disease Patients and their Social Needs*. Parkinson's Disease Society, London.

Parkes, J.D. (1982). *Parkinson's Disease*. Update Postgraduate Series. Update Publications Ltd., London.

Sacks, O. (1973). *Awakenings*. Duckworth & Co., London.

Scott, S., and Caird, F.I. (1983). Speech therapy for Parkinson's disease. *Journal of Neurology, Neurosurgery and Psychiatry, 46,* 140-4.

Singer, E. (1972). Social costs of Parkinson's disease. *Journal of Chronic Diseases, 24, 4,* 243-52.

5 METHODS OF ASSESSMENT OF THE SPEECH DISORDER OF PARKINSON'S DISEASE

There is a lack of objective documentation of the management of dysarthria and of the efficacy of therapy and this is linked with a lack of standardised assessment techniques. As the incidence of acquired dysarthria is high, it is surprising that so few speech therapists have looked for ways of assessing its effect upon speech. There are many reliable methods of assessment of disorders of language but no standardised method is universally available for assessing disturbances of the speaker's characteristics of voice and dynamics (Laver, 1981). Current research is attempting to remedy this situation.

Assessment can be perceptual, instrumental or both. Perceptual evaluation is based on the clinician judging samples of the subject's voice, best recorded on tape. Such judgments customarily rely on impressionistic terms of description which may not be reproducible or be capable of reliable translation. In the past observations were based upon acoustic assessment of oral reading tests such as Fairbanks' 'Rainbow Passage'. Such phonetically balanced tests formed the basis of Canter's (1963, 1965a, b) studies.

Instrumental assessment enables a more objective approach to the evaluation of speech parameters. It utilises such techniques as electrolaryngography, xeroradiography, spectrographic studies and spirometry, all of which allow the examination of the speech functions of the vocal tract with considerable accuracy. They are generally considered to be unsuitable techniques for everyday clinical use, both because of their cost and because of the time needed for training therapists in their application. Therefore therapists have to rely on a perceptual evaluation, whatever the shortcomings of such a system. Errors can occur no matter how experienced the speech therapist, and concomitant factors (see Chapter 3) will affect speech performance. In addition, particularly in the case of Parkinson's disease, speech intelligibility need not correlate with the degree of motor impairment observed in the speech musculature or with the acoustic description of speech production and speech function at a single word or single phrase level (Sarno, 1968). It is therefore not representative of the degree of conversational dysfunction.

Speech therapists need to assess a motor speech disorder objectively in order to determine the nature and degree of difficulty present and the most appropriate therapeutic method available. In severe cases of Parkinson's disease it is important to remember that the reduced verbal flow and general muscle immobility may make assessment almost impossible.

The use of Proprioceptive Neuromuscular Facilitation (PNF) assessment techniques (Table 5.1) may be of value in such severe cases. This is particularly so in the management of swallowing difficulties, where in many cases such assessment is a pre-cursor to treatment, serving as preparation for movement in cases presenting with a reduction of sensation and lip seal.

In the most severe cases one must also assess for the suitability of a non-verbal method of communication (see Chapter 8).

Perceptual Methods of Assessment

The most commonly used perceptual method is the check list or rating scale. Thompson (1978) outlined a specific rating scale for Parkinson's disease but stressed that it is subject to the limitations of all such methods. The use of the scale requires a special degree of experience on the part of the therapist in the management of Parkinson's disease. It takes into account the individual and variable speech dysfunctions of Parkinson's disease, and the complex nature of their interaction. It is however arbitrary and may place undue emphasis upon vocal features inappropriately. Thompson (1978) has described eight speech dimensions which are characteristically disturbed in Parkinson's disease and which require assessment (Table 5.2).

A similar rating scale was used by Scott and Caird (1981, 1983) for prosodic abnormality (Table 5.3). Respiratory and articulatory function were also included in this assessment, but it was noted that it was the degree of prosodic abnormality that mainly influenced speech intelligibility. Assessment was concentrated on seven speech functions found to be disturbed in Parkinson's disease. The samples of recorded speech taken during the assessments were analysed independently by a second speech therapist. The high degree of reproducibility (Figure 5.1) achieved indicated that there

Table 5.1: PNF Checklist of the Organs of Articulation and Respiration

		Features examined	Comments
1.	Head and neck movements	Range of mobility Control	
2.	Breathing	Symmetry of muscular activity Extent of intercostal function Extent of diaphragmatic function Control of inspiration	
3.	Phonation	Vocal cord function (CN *X*)	
	Reflex phonatory function	Coughing (CN *V,X*)	

4.	Swallowing and sucking
	    muscle:
	        Range
	        Symmetry
	        Force
		Orbicularis oris CN *VII*
		Buccinator CN *VII*
		Tongue CN *XII*
		Soft palate CN *V,X*	

5.	Facial musculature
	    muscle:
	        Range
	        Symmetry
	        Force
		Frontalis
		Corrugator
		Orbicularis occuli
		Nasalis
		Levator labii sup. alaeque
		    nasi
		Zygomaticus
		Depressor anguli oris
		Levator labii anguli
		Buccinator
		Risorius	

6.	Muscles of mastication
	    muscle:
	        Rate
	        Symmetry
	        Force
		Temporalis
		Masseter
		Pterygoids
		Orbicularis oris
		Buccinator	

Source: Scott and Caird (1981).

would be little difficulty in its use for speech therapists who had been trained to appreciate the various effects of prosody upon speech and in particular those features disturbed by Parkinson's disease. The scale is specific to prosodic abnormality, and focuses attention on the suprasegmental aspects of speech. Recent work by

Table 5.2: Parkinson's Disease Speech Rating Scale

Emotional behaviour

Congruent	Confused	Lethargic
Depressed	Euphoric	Labile
Anxious	Unco-operative	
Other		

Saliva in mouth

Excessive	Normal	Reduced
Effect on speech		

Intensity
   0 — No impairment.
   1 — Overall speech intensity slightly reduced.
   2 — Overall intensity moderately below the normal range. Weak vocalisation still audible.
   3 — Speech aphonic.

Speech decay
   0 — No impairment.
   1 — Mild decay of vocal intensity and articulatory contact at the end of speech segments.
   2 — Moderate reduction in vocal intensity and articulatory contact at the end of segments.
   3 — Speech decay severe. Word endings frequently unintelligible owing to poor articulatory contact. Weak/absent vocalisation.

Vocal quality
   0 — No impairment.
     (i)   Constant:
     1 — Slightly hoarse quality superimposed on entire speech flow.
     2 — Moderate hoarse quality.
     3 — Forced, hoarse quality. Visible effort expended in vocalising.
                            OR
     (ii) Fluctuating:
     1 — Occasional fluctuation in vocal fold quality resulting in moments of hoarse quality interspersed in a speech flow of normal vocal quality.
     2 — Approximately 50 per cent of the speech flow is produced with normal quality. Hoarse quality interspersed randomly over words, phrases or sentences.
     3 — Hoarse quality predominates, but moments of normal vocal quality are still detectable in the speech flow.

Prosody
   0 — No impairment.
   1 — Slight dysprosody. Speech slightly monotonous.
   2 — Speech monotony pronounced, but some use of stress and inflection still evident.
   3 — Severe dysprosody. Speech produced in a flat, unvarying monotone.

Source: Modified after Thompson (1978).

Table 5 3: Prosodic Abnormality Score

A.	Volume	Loud
		Mono
		Normal
		Quiet
		Fading
B.	Pitch	High
		Low
		Normal
		Monotone
		Breaks
C.	Tone	Hyper
		Mixed
		Normal
		Hypo
D.	Intonation	Monotone
		Reduced
		Normal
		Inappropriate
E.	Vocal quality	Hoarse
		Strident
		Normal
		Tremor
		Aphonic
F.	Rate	Too fast
		Progressively increasing in speed
		Normal
		Progressively decreasing in speed
		Slow
G.	Rhythm	Stammerlike
		Insufficient stressing
		Normal
		Inappropriate silences

Normal: Score 0 on each item A–G
Any abnormality: Score 1 on each item A–G
Maximum score: 7

Source: Scott and Caird (1981).

Laver (1983) has further demonstrated the reliability of the prosodic abnormality score which correlates well with computer speech analysis of the tapes. It may be that, in future, methods such as computer voice analysis and soft tissue xeroradiography may form the basis of a central bank to which therapists might send tapes for more comprehensive analysis. This could overcome the prohibitive costs of the use of such instrumental techniques in

Figure 5.1: Prosodic Abnormality Scores Obtained from Analysis of Speech Tapes by Two Therapists Independently: 110 Tapes were Analysed — 15 Per Cent (16) Differed, None by More than One Point

	Observer 1: Prosodic Abnormality Score							
Observer 2: Prosodic Abnormality Score	0	1	2	3	4	5	6	7
0								
1		3	[3]					
2		[1]	15	[1]				
3				15	[1]			
4					20	[6]		
5					[3]	16		
6						[1]	13	
7								9

normal clinical practice, and could enable therapists to use the valuable objective analyses which result from them as a means on which to base therapy.

Proprioceptive Neuromuscular Facilitation and Dysarthria Assessments

Therapists are required to assess the range of movement of the organs of articulation. A short and practical method might be the form used by exponents of Proprioceptive Neuromuscular Facilitation (PNF) — see Table 5.1.

The examination of the symmetry and range of specific facial muscles provides the groundwork for movement and increases the sensory awareness of the mouth in preparation for therapy. It is particularly useful in determining the nature and extent of swallowing difficulties and the degree of impoverished facial expression.

The use of PNF techniques has been shown to be effective in the management of the speech disorder of Parkinson's disease (Scott and Caird, 1981).

More recently the development of a new dysarthria assessment by Enderby (1980), offering a profile of function in areas of reflex activity, particularly respiration, lips, jaw, palate, laryngeal and tongue areas, would appear to offer therapists a more objective mode of assessment. Although it is not specific to Parkinson's

Table 5 4: Test for Receptive Speech Difficulty

Test 1: Discrimination of prosodic contrasts.
In all the examples (except h) responses are made to prosodic rather than to phonemic contrasts. The phrases were presented in pairs (i.e. a neutral statement with another example) and the subjects commented on whether these pairs were the same or different.
The following phrases were played on tape:
a.   I can run. (neutral statement)
b.   I can run. (emphatic stress on *run*)
c.   I can run. (emphatic stress on *can*)
d.   I can run. (neutral statement)
e.   I can run. (exaggerated pause between can and run)
f.   I can. Run! (double phrase; statement and command)
g.   I can run? (intonational form of interrogative style of phrase)
h.   Can I run? (differing interrogative word order)
The maximum possible score was 8.

Test 2: Matching of speech and facial expression.
Patients were asked to describe each of the facial expressions shown in the cartoons in Figure 2.1, and thereafter listened to a taped phrase and selected the most appropriate facial expression to the single taped phrase. The maximum score was 1.

Test 3: Discrimination of the affective and grammatical functions of prosody.
Subjects listened to the following sentences on tape and commented upon the emotional features presented.
a.   It's me, Alison. (nominative function, i.e. 'me' and 'Alison' in apposition)
b.   It's me, Alison. (vocative function, i.e. 'me' and 'Alison' as different people)
c.   Don't hurry. (sarcasm)
d.   Don't hurry. (caring advice)
e.   Good morning. (officious and abrupt greeting)
f.   Good morning. (pleasant greeting)
g.   I scream. (the action)*
h.   Ice-cream. (the confection)*
*Demonstrates a grammatical function of prosody.
The maximum possible score was 8.

Test 4: Discrimination of the semantic role of prosody.
Subjects had to comment on whether the paired phrases in Test 1, had the same or different meanings. The maximum possible score was 4.

Test 5: Production of anger.
Subjects were asked to read the following sentences in an angry tone of voice:
a.   I don't want to go.
b.   That's my pen.
c.   Go away.
The maximum score was 3.

Test 6: Production of question form.
The subjects were asked to produce the same phrases as in Test 5 in a questioning or doubtful manner. The maximum score was 3.

Test 7: Production of statement form.
Subjects were asked to read the phrases in Test 5, as neutral statements. The maximum score was 3.

disease, Enderby's current studies should validate the dysarthria assessment in the elderly.

The current work of Robertson and Thomson (1984) may provide a formal method of clinical assessment of dysarthria which will allow the therapist to interpret the patient's vocal and speech weaknesses and strengths. The use of this assessment technique in the management of Parkinson's disease affords the therapist an excellent clinical tool upon which treatment techniques may be based.

The recent studies of Scott *et al.* (1984) have indicated that each patient should be assessed to determine the presence of an underlying perceptual prosodic difficulty. The specific method of assessment for this perceptual element in Parkinson's disease is shown in Table 5.4.

It is necessary to exclude several other specific influences upon speech, as mentioned in Chapter 3, particularly prior to determining the presence or absence of a sensory or perceptual difficulty. Problems of auditory discrimination, hearing loss, language abnormality, and particularly dementia influence the features of speech which generate stress, intonation, affective speech, and volume and pitch variation.

In her recent investigation of the communication status of the elderly, Walker (1982) suggested that linguistic analyses of spontaneous and test-elicited speech reveal that discrete qualitative changes and combinations of these changes, in particular the presence of phonemic naming errors, single element utterances (e.g. house) and failure on a ten selected item naming task from section C11 of the Minnesota Test for the Differential Diagnosis of Aphasia (Schuell *et al.*, 1968), were differentiating features of dementia. Screening Parkinson patient's with the above should detect subjects with a specific language difficulty or dementia. The presence of moderately severe dementia may influence several linguistic features of a patient and should assessment indicate its presence, prosodic therapy is not indicated.

References

Canter, G.J. (1963). Speech characteristics of patients with Parkinson's disease. I. Intensity, pitch and duration. *Journal of*

Speech and Hearing Disorders, 28, 221-9.

_____ (1965a). Speech characteristics of patients with Parkinson's disease. II. Physiological support for speech. *Journal of Speech and Hearing Disorders, 30,* 44-9.

_____ (1965b). Speech characteristics of patients with Parkinson's disease. III. Articulation diadochonkinesis, and overall speech adequacy. *Journal of Speech and Hearing Disorders, 30,* 217-24.

Darley, F.L., Aronson, A.E., and Brown, J.R. (1975). *Motor Speech Disorders.* W.B. Saunders Co., Philadelphia.

Enderby, P. (1980). Frenchay Dysarthria Assessment. *British Journal of Disorders of Communication, 15,* 165-73.

Fairbanks, G. (1960). *Voice and Articulation Drill Book,* Harper & Row, 2nd edn. New York.

Laver, J. (1981). *Phonetic Description of Voice Quality.* Cambridge University Press, Cambridge.

_____ (1983). Paper presented at IALP Conference, Edinburgh.

Peacher, W.G. (1949). Etiology and differential diagnosis of dysarthria. *Journal of Speech and Hearing Disorders, 15,* 252-65.

Powell, G., Clark, E., and Bailey, S. (1978). A very short version of the Minnesota aphasia test. *British Journal of Social Psychology, 19,* 189-94.

Robertson, S., and Thomson, F. (1984). Speech therapy in Parkinson's disease. A study of the efficacy and long-term effects of intensive speech therapy. *British Journal of Disorders of Communication* (in press).

Sarno, M.T. (1968). Speech impairment in Parkinson's disease. *Archives of Physical Medicine and Rehabilitation, 49,* 269-75.

Scott, S., and Caird, F.I. (1981). Speech therapy for patients with Parkinson's disease. *British Medical Journal, 283,* 1088.

_____ (1983). Speech therapy for Parkinson's disease. *Journal of Neurology, Neurosurgery and Psychiatry, 46,* 140-4.

Scott, S., Caird, F.I., and Williams, B.O. (1984). Evidence for an apparent sensory disorder in Parkinson's disease. *Journal of Neurology, Neurosurgery and Psychiatry* (in press).

Thompson, A.K. (1978). A clinical rating scale for speech dysfunction in Parkinson's disease. *South African Journal of Communication Disorders, 25,* 39-52.

Walker, S.A. (1982). Investigation of the communication of elderly subjects. MPhil thesis, University of Leicester.

6 DRUG THERAPY AND ITS EFFECT ON SPEECH IN THE PARKINSONIAN PATIENT

In the drug management of Parkinsonism (Table 6.1) the belladonna alkaloids were originally given as plant extracts in mixtures, tinctures or smoked with tobacco. In the last 25 years or more a range of synthetic agents have been prescribed as 'anticholinergic preparations'. These will usually slightly improve the Parkinsonian patient by producing a slight reduction in tremor and rigidity. No single anticholinergic preparation is more efficacious than another, while with all of them side-effects can be very troublesome, especially in the elderly (Table 6.2).

Table 6 1: Drug Management of Parkinsonism

Mild	symptoms but no disability	1 anticholinergics (Artane, etc.) 2 amantadine (Symmetrel)
Moderate	disabled but independent	1 levodopa/decarboxylase inhibitor combination (Sinemet or Madopar) 2 anticholinergics
Severe	dependent	1 Sinemet or Madopar 2 bromocriptine (Parlodel) 3 pergolide 4 lisuride 5 selegiline (Eldepryl)

Table 6 2: Side-effects of Anticholinergic Drugs

Central	Confusion Hallucinations
Peripheral	Dryness of mouth Blurring of vision Constipation Retention of urine

The much greater effectiveness of levodopa in the treatment of Parkinsonism has been well demonstrated, and there has been a slight resultant increase in the life expectancy of patients with this disorder. Combination therapy with levodopa and a peripheral dopadecarboxylase inhibitor, such as carbidopa or benserazide, has been shown to have greater efficacy and fewer side-effects than levodopa alone (Table 6.3). A combination preparation is thus now the first choice in those patients in whom levodopa therapy is indicated, i.e. when the disabilities present compromise independence. Disability and symptoms are alleviated for several years, but the natural course of the disease is unaltered.

More recent advances in antiparkinson therapy include the introduction of bromocriptine, pergolide, lisuride and selegiline. These drugs may have a useful role as replacements for and adjuvants to levodopa therapy, but again, side-effects may limit their use (Table 6.4).

Drug therapy is probably the most important part of the rehabilitation of the Parkinsonian patient. If appropriate it will transform the patient's existence, but if inappropriate it can lead to grave and occasionally irremediable loss of independence.

What constitutes appropriate drug treatment depends on the clinical features of the disease in the individual case. In general levodopa preparations are indicated if there is significant bradykinesia

Table 6 3: Side-effects of Levodopa Preparations

Central	Confusion
	Depression
	Hypomania
	Dyskinesia
	On/off attacks
Peripheral	Hypotension
	Nausea and vomiting

Table 6 4: Side-effects of Bromocriptine

Confusion
Sedation
Nausea and vomiting
Dyskinesia

or rigidity and anticholinergic drugs such as benzhexol and benztropine, or levodopa, if tremor is a problem. Beta-blocking drugs such as propranolol may be useful in some cases of tremor, but their effects are unpredictable, presumably because the underlying mechanisms of tremor are multiple. In general they are of minimal value in extrapyramidal tremor.

Mental state is the most significant determinant of the response to levodopa in affected patients. If intellectual impairment is absent or slight, the prognosis for treatment is good, but if there is severe impairment, drug treatment rarely produces much benefit, and all too often exacerbates the psychiatric disorder. Mild extrapyramidal signs are often encountered in elderly patients with non-vascular or vascular forms of dementia. These patients are not suffering from Parkinson's disease and they very rarely benefit from drug treatment and may be made much worse by it.

Levodopa treatment should begin with small doses and only small increments should be made, initially at intervals of five days or more. Anticholinergic drugs should not usually be given until the apparent optimal dose of levodopa has been reached and even then only in patients who have troublesome tremor. Drug regimens should always be kept as simple as possible.

The earliest therapeutic effects of levodopa include an increase in the strength of the voice, followed by increased mobility consequent to reduction in rigidity and bradykinesia. Side-effects (Table 6.5) include orofacial dyskinesia and orthostatic hypotension. Both may indicate the need for a small reduction in daily levodopa dosage, but minor dyskinesias may have to be accepted. Orthostatic hypotension is usually asymptomatic and resolves in a few weeks, except if it is a late side-effect.

Table 6.5: Drugs Which May Adversely Affect Speech in Parkinson's Disease

benzodiazepines
tricyclic antidepressants
phenothiazines
lithium
anticonvulsants
anticholinergics
levodopa (peak dosage)
alcohol

Seventy per cent of patients with Parkinson's disease derive some benefit from treatment with levodopa, and in half the improvement may be substantial. It is becoming clear however that with continued levodopa therapy there is a decline in benefit over a two to five year period; more and more patients develop what is termed late drug failure, which is either side-effects of the drug or manifestations of later stages of the natural history of the disease.

Thus various dyskinetic movements may occur and they may vary with time after each dose. This is due to either a presumed peak effect of each dose of levodopa, or at the end of the effectiveness of each dose. The so-called 'on-off' phenomenon is manifest by rapid fluctuations in the patient's physical abilities (including speech) occurring over periods of minutes, during which the patient may change from reasonable mobility to total immobility, and then back again.

The Effect of Drugs upon Speech

Before 1970, there were few reports about the effects of drugs or surgical intervention on the speech disorder of Parkinsonian patients, in part because speech involvement was a contraindication to surgery. Speech did not seem to be improved by anticholinergic drugs or surgery. The introduction of levodopa changed the situation. Rigrodsky and Morrison (1970) assessed the effect on oral communication of maximal dosage of levodopa in 21 patients with Parkinson's disease. Speech improvement was not thought to be as dramatic as the general physical improvement achieved. Oral reading and spontaneous speech appeared to improve during the first four weeks of therapy. However, although there was improvement in terms of overall adequacy, clarity of articulation and 'normalcy' of nasal resonance, it was only in the rate of speech that statistically significant change was observed. Mawdsley and Gamsu (1971) observed that levodopa effectively improved speech intelligibility in most patients. They noted an increase in voice volume and a reduction in dysarthria. The rate of speech did not alter, but during therapy each phoneme took a significantly shorter time to utter and was separated from the preceding and following phonemes by lengthened pauses. There was a tendency for both phonation and pauses to be more regularly distributed after treatment. The resultant shorter and crisper sounds were separated by better defined pauses; this improved the clarity of speech.

Wolfe *et al.* (1975) confirmed that levodopa did not affect the rate of speech production, but they also observed significant improvement in voice quality, pitch variation and articulation. They considered that the degree of speech changes correlated well with the amount of physical improvement and observed that speech improvement can occur whatever the age of the patient or the duration of the disease. In this, the first report of longer-term levodopa effects, three of a total of four patients manifested further improvement in speech or maintained their state after four years of drug treatment.

Electromyographic studies of the labial musculature have shown that Parkinsonian patients with speech disorders have constant abnormally increased tonic activity, and a systematic disturbance of reciprocal muscular activation. Levodopa normalises the electromyographic pattern and can re-establish reciprocal inhibition of the antagonists in their articulatory muscles. The latency between initiation of labial movement and speech is shortened, and the speed and symmetry of labial activity is increased (Nakano *et al.*, 1973).

Voice production in the Parkinsonian patient depends both on respiratory control and on mental state. Levodopa may perhaps act not only on peripheral articulatory and phonatory mechanisms, but also on higher mental function to improve overall speech ability.

Adverse Effects of Drugs upon Speech

A number of drugs often given to Parkinson's disease patients may adversely affect their speech (Table 6.1). In patients whose levodopa dosage has been too high and who develop orofacial dyskinesia, speech may become unintelligible due to akinesia and dysphonia at the peak of levodopa action (Marsden and Parkes, 1976; Critchley, 1976).

Drugs may compromise the higher functions which determine the content of speech or they may alter the form and articulatory precision of speech. The review by Gawel (1981) is comprehensive on this subject. The benzodiazepines, e.g. diazepam or nitrazepam, in large doses may produce slurring of speech and even in therapeutic doses may adversely affect higher integrative functions. This may result in the increased utterance of remarks which are often not understandable or are inaudible. Sentences and phrases tend to be incomplete.

The tricyclic antidepressants, e.g. amitriptyline or imipramine, may promote speech blockage in which the patient has difficulty in expressing a word; this may result in the punctuation of otherwise normal speech patterns with prolonged pauses. The central anticholinergic effects of these compounds may adversely affect higher cortical functions and produce dysarthria. The side-effects of the phenothiazines, e.g. thioridazine or chlorpromazine, include tardive dyskinesia in which orofacial writhing movements and dysarthria occur. Lithium may cause dysarthria, while cerebellar dysarthria may occur as a side effect of anticonvulsant medication, e.g. phenytoin.

References

Critchley, E.M.R. (1976). Peak-dose dysphonia in Parkinsonism. *Lancet, 1,* 544.

Gawel, M.J. (1981). The effects of various drugs on speech. *British Journal of Disorders of Communication, 16,* 51-7.

Leanderson, R., Meyerson, B.A., and Persson, A. (1971). Effect of L-dopa on speech in Parkinsonism. *Journal of Neurology, Neurosurgery and Psychiatry, 34,* 679-81.

Marsden, C.D., and Parkes, J.D. (1976). 'On-off' effects on patients with Parkinson's disease on chronic levodopa therapy. *Lancet, 1,* 292-6.

Mawdsley, C., and Gamsu, C.V. (1971). Periodicity of speech in Parkinsonism. *Nature, 231,* 315-6.

Nakano, K.K., Kubick, H., and Tyler, H.R. (1973). Speech defects of Parkinsonian patients. Effects of levodopa therapy on speech intelligibility. *Neurology, 23,* 865-70.

Perry, A.R., and Das, P.K. (1981). Speech assessment of patients with Parkinson's disease. In Rose, F.C., and Capildeo, R. (eds), *Progress in Parkinson's Disease,* Pitman Medical, London, pp. 373-84.

Rigrodsky, S., and Morrison, E.B. (1970). Speech changes in Parkin-

sonism during L-dopa therapy: preliminary findings. *Journal of the American Geriatrics Society, 18*, 142-51.
Wolfe, V.I., Garvin, J.S., Bacon, M., and Waldrop, W. (1975). Speech changes in Parkinson's disease during treatment with L-dopa. *Journal of Communication Disorders, 8*, 271-9.

7 THE EFFECT OF SPEECH THERAPY UPON COMMUNICATION

In general speech therapy for the Parkinson's disease sufferer is aimed at maximising the patient's available functioning speech. Many authors regard therapy as the restoration of muscular activity through exercise, or the facilitation of sensory responses to stimulate a motor reaction, e.g. with vibration, electric stimulation, or stroking with ice (Draper, 1968; Greene, 1980), or as encompassing phonemic drills aimed at achieving precise articulation and thus restoring functional speech.

Traditionally speech treatment in degenerative disorders has been discouraged (Peacher, 1947). Opinions have differed about the appropriateness of therapy in such situations. Treatment was considered as either unrealistic or as a life-long obligation for the therapist (Allan, 1970), or that it might alter the sufferer's psyche but not his speech intelligibility (Sarno, 1968). The role of the speech therapist in Parkinson's disease was that of assessor during periods of hospital admission for drug titration or pre- and post-operatively (Greene, 1980). These views and the progressive nature of Parkinson's disease discouraged many therapists. Referrals from doctors for therapeutic intervention were rare, as they preferred to rely solely on the effects of medication. This attitude was also adopted by speech therapists (Perry, 1981).

Traditional Methods of Treatment

Early communication treatment has, however, been advocated by some as a means of retarding the inevitable degeneration of function in more slowly progressive disorders such as Parkinsonism (Darley *et al.*, 1975; Morley, 1955).

Calne (1970) considered that the best results of speech therapy occurred in patients who were medically stable and in whom speech improvement had already occurred as a response to drugs. Despite otherwise optimal drug treatments however, obvious speech abnormality may persist. Rosenbek and La Pointe (1978) believed that it is with the failed medical case that therapists should try hardest, and similarly with patients in whom surgical intervention techniques have aggravated speech difficulties. Scott and Caird (1983) have recently argued the value of speech therapy in all cases with speech disorder.

Coexisting intellectual deterioration, psychiatric disturbance, hearing loss and dysphasia are most important influences on decisions regarding treatment (see Chapter 3), because speech therapy usually requires active patient participation (Rosenbek and La Pointe, 1978).

Until recently the efficacy and benefits of therapy were rarely analysed objectively. Greene and Watson (1968) considered that the loss of volume was the most responsive to therapy, stressing relaxation and reassurance to maintain a good standard of speech performance, and inspiring a patient to make the best use of residual function. Butfield (1961) emphasised the therapist's role in encouragement to keep alive the patient's desire to communicate.

Canter (1963) made an extensive examination of various speech parameters in Parkinson's disease and concluded that previous 'negative' opinions towards therapy were unjustified. Teaching patients to make the most of their limited speech ability seemed inappropriate when they were capable of better performance.

Early methods of therapy are summarised in Table 7.1 and they include many adapted from traditional voice therapy, e.g. forcing exercises recommended by Butfield (1961) to obtain better abduction of the laryngeal folds (Table 7.2). This approach was similar to that of Froeschel (1948) who stressed the importance of synchrony between the pushing action and phonation. However, it can be argued that such an energetic technique is inappropriate with an elderly person and that it tends to cause speech to occur on held inspiration, or that it promotes speech flow on end-phase expiration. Both these latter features are already present in the voicing of Parkinson's disease.

Techniques to alter pitch and improve vocal function have been encouraged, for example the chewing therapy of Froeschel (1948) and Smith's (1951) techniques of relaxation, flowing movement and vocalisation.

Mechanical Aids

Greene and Watson (1968) introduced amplification devices to

Table 7.1: Traditional Methods of Therapy

Method	Method Aim	Technique
Chewing therapy (Froeschel, 1948)	Improving voicing, correct pitch placement	Chewing savagely while simultaneously voicing
Eurythmic approach (Smith, 1951)	Improving breathing, improving voicing	Relaxed total body movements in rhythmic sequences during vocalisation
Forcing exercises (Butfield, 1961)	Improving vocal fold adduction	Synchronised pushing with voicing
Syllabic speech (Andrews & Harris, 1964)	Reduce tension, improve speech rhythm	Speech is timed to a slow and regular tapped beat at the start of syllable
Amplification (Green & Watson, 1968)	Reduce tension, increase voice volume mechanically	Patient's voice is amplified by a mechanical aid
Metronome therapy (Wohl, 1968)	Improve speech rhythm, improve voice onset	Syllable timed speech using a metronome aid
Group therapy (Allan, 1970)	Improve voicing rate and clarity	Group practice of selected articulation exercises, speech phrases and conversation practice

Table 7 2: Forcing Exercises Recommended by Butfield (1961)

1. Laugh or cough; thereafter endeavour to prolong the spasmodic phonation thus achieved into a protracted vowel.
2. Swallow and phonate [i:].
3. Link the fingers, lift arms to the level of the clavicle and pull against each other, phonating on [i:].
4. Push hands against a table and phonate as before.

alleviate problems of vocal failure. They considered that the most important function of the amplifier was to reduce tension and anxiety, which may arise through the patient's fear of being inaudible. Voice is raised as a natural reaction to background noise (Lombard effect). When too quiet speech is amplified a patient will automatically continue to match speech with the amplified output for some time after the latter has been switched off (Greene, 1980). Such devices are useful in cases where loss of volume is the only disorder of communication. The aid merely amplifies already aberrant aspects of speech; it may also prove awkward for the elderly to operate alone. As with many electronic aids the value is individual and to be useful they require considerable persistence on the part of the user. They are however useful adjuncts to therapy, and serve as a means of self-monitoring. Cooper-Rand have recently introduced a 'no hands' amplifier which makes it a more useful therapeutic aid. Amplification is most valuable in cases where spouses have hearing loss, or when the short-term effects of voice amplification are required for business meetings. Another valuable amplification device in Britain is supplied by British Telecom; it is fitted to the telephone and amplifies the voice of the user. Greene (1981) has advocated that amplification appears on the whole to be the most promising and logical approach to the Parkinson patient's speech problem, but in our opinion this has not been proven satisfactorily.

The use of electronic metronomes has been advocated for the treatment of festinant speech by Wohl (1968) and Allan (1970). The rhythmical pulse or, if not available, the manual tapping, regulates the pattern of speech flow. Allan stressed that the patient must be well preserved mentally to derive benefit from such techniques. The elderly, and more advanced cases of Parkinson's disease, find the procedures confusing. A similar technique utilising syllabic speech has been considered (Andrews and Harris, 1964), but found to have little lasting value outside the clinic, since patients fail to grasp its significance.

A loudness level meter on a tape recorder to aid monitoring and control of volume fluctuations has been recommended (Perry and Das, 1981).

More recent methods of therapy are summarised in Table 7.3. Helm (1979) utilised a pacing board with one Parkinson's disease patient. She considered this to be a practical application of Luria's (1967) theory; motor acts can be transferred to a cortical level by substituting a series of individual conscious impulses for a patterned response cycle. This is a method often utilised by physiotherapists to facilitate more normal walking patterns. Helm found that the pacing board was a useful therapeutic aid in controlling palilalia: patients feel along the board as they speak, and, in conformity with Luria's theory of intersystemic reorganisation, the physical barrier encountered influences the speech flow. The application is limited, however, and the question remains as to whether the patient will require the board permanently to maintain functional speech. No further studies have been documented, although

Table 7.3: Recent Methods of Therapy

Method	Method Aim	Technique	Timing
Pacing board (Helm, 1979, after Luria)	Reduce rate, inhibit initiation difficulties	patient feels along a stepped board; the physical barrier met by the hand is transferred into speech	Particularly useful in clinic for rate control
Delayed Auditory Feedback (Downie *et al.*, 1981)	Reduce rate, overcome onset difficulties	Mechanical feedback masks the patient's speech, causing reduced rate and sound prolongation	Limited use
Proprioceptive Neuromuscular Facilitation (Scott & Caird, 1981)	Improve facial expression, voice intensity, respiration and swallowing	Specific manipulation of muscles	Very useful technique at all stages of the disease process
Prosodic therapy (Scott & Caird, 1983)	Improve rate rhythm, intonation, vocal expression, vocal intensity	Exercises emphasising the affective and prosodic aspects of speech	Very useful at all stages of the disease process, except at end stage of the disease
Residential holiday therapy (Robertson & Thompson, 1984)	Social and conversational improvement	Intensive group therapy	Useful for mild and moderately handicapped sufferers

Rosenbek and La Pointe (1978) have developed several variations such as button-pushing and ball-squeezing. One might consider the tapping and metronome techniques as similar manners of production in such reorganisation.

Delayed Auditory Feedback (DAF) techniques have recently been considered to be successful methods of management. Rosenbek and La Pointe (1978) tentatively suggested that DAF influences articulation time and adequacy. A delay interval of 50 milliseconds has been shown to have a beneficial effect upon prosody, but delays of 100 milliseconds or more have detrimental effects upon the dysarthric speaker. Similarly the effects vary, depending upon the stimuli used. The technique has been found to be less effective in propositional speech. Rosenbek and La Pointe further advocated its use as part of behavioural therapy, the aim being to wean the patient from the machine. Its use is most convincing in demonstrating to the patient that dramatic speech improvement is possible. Downie *et al.*, (1981) noted marked improvement in the speech intelligibility of two 'festinant' patients using DAF, but considered that the aid would have to be used permanently in order to maintain the level of functional competence achieved.

In Britain a new form of electronic aid, the Royal National Institute for the Deaf (RNID) 'Visispeech' unit, has recently been introduced as a possible feedback device for patients with 'dysprosodic' speech. This system can be combined with an adaptation of the Apple computer and allows the therapist to set vocal patterns of stressing and intonation upon the computer screen, in order that the patient might copy them and compare their performance with that of the therapist. It provides disc storage and hard copy records of the therapy session. It is not unlike the 'Visipitch' instrument, which provides visual representations of the voice characteristics of pitch, voice onset, vocal quality and intonation.

These computerised units are useful in the initial assessment and diagnosis of patients and as individual therapy session aids, or for record purposes. The 'Visispeech' also has an eight-track output on a visual display unit and can therefore be incorporated in a group treatment session or model shorter conversational sessions.

Traditional attempts to facilitate adequate palatropharyngeal closure in order to achieve resonant speech are singularly ineffective. The usual techniques of blowing and sucking are now considered to be aimed at palatopharyngeal functions other than those of speech and do not significantly alter the palatopharyngeal gap (Powers and Starr, 1974). Selley and Tudor (1974) advocated the fitting of a prosthetic lift to dentures (Palatal Aid) to improve speech, increase resonance, facilitate swallowing and improve eating habits. The use of the aid has been noted to inhibit excessive salivation. Similarly the fitting of sulcus eliminator aids, advocated in dysphasic patients, has been found to improve the retention of dentures and facilitate mastication. Our experience is that the increased buccal padding of the sulcus eliminator is most valuable, but the palatal lift is poorly tolerated and not to be recommended in cases of severe tremor.

PNF and Prosodic Therapy

A pilot study (Scott and Caird, 1981) led to the evaluation of remedial techniques which may be more appropriate. A comparison was made between a physical method of therapy (PNF: Proprioceptive Neuromuscular Facilitation) and a method emphasising the prosodic aspects alone (this utilised prosodic exercises). Treatment with prosodic exercises aimed at increasing the patient's awareness of the abnormal prosodic features in his own speech and encouraged practice in more normal patterns of conversational speech. This was supplemented by a voice-operated visual reinforcement device, the Vocalite (Figure 7.1).

PNF proved valuable in establishing pursed lip breathing, whereby the subject's awareness of breathing was reduced and relaxed expiratory phases reinforced. It was also invaluable in establishing the correct body and lip postures for speech, in inhibiting drooling and in facilitating swallowing. This technique is effective but requires intensive training of the therapist, whereas the prosodic exercise method may be more practical in clinical terms. A formal trial was then established to evaluate the effects of this latter method (Scott and Caird, 1983).

Twenty-six patients with the speech disorder of Parkinson's disease received daily prosodic exercise therapy at home for two weeks (Group A) or three weeks (Group B). The patients were

Figure 7.1: The Vocalite, a Voice-operated Visual Reinforcement Device

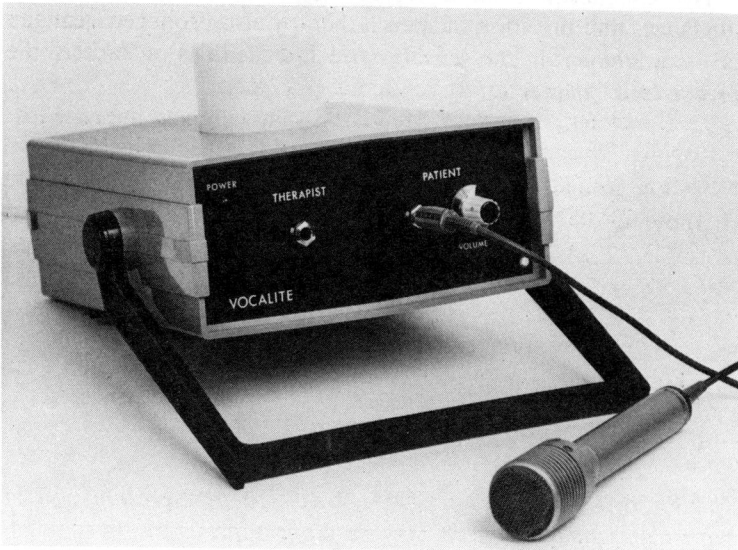

representative of those with the speech disorder of Parkinson's disease in respect of age, duration of the disease and drug therapy.

There was significant improvement in speech production and, in addition, increased awareness of the prosodic features in the speech of others. This improvement was maintained in part for up to three months (Table 7.4 and Figure 7.2). There was not only an improvement in scores, as relatives commented on the practical and social benefits gained (see Table 4.1). Small changes in prosodic abnormality could in individual patients be associated with substantial improvement in social communication. The use of the visual reinforcement device produced limited benefit over and above that of exercise alone, except among those patients with severe speech disorders.

An analysis of the effects of therapy on the individual features making up the prosodic abnormality score showed that they could be divided into three groups. Abnormality of intonation and rhythm were universally present and improved only marginally. Abnormalities of vocal quality, rate and volume were present in 80 per cent of patients and improved substantially; and this improvement was largely maintained. Abnormalities of pitch and tone were present in 50 per cent or fewer, and showed some improvement, but this was not well maintained in assessment number 5 (Table 7.5 and Figure 7.3).

The conclusion from a subsequent study (Scott and Caird, 1984) was that this form of speech therapy also produced substantial improvement in the sensory speech difficulties of Parkinson's disease (see Chapter 2).

Table 7.4: Mean Prosodic Abnormality Score before and after Therapy

| | | Assessment Number | | |
| | Before therapy began | 2 weeks therapy with vocalite (Group A) without vocalite (Group B) | 1 week additional therapy with vocalite (Group B only) | 3 month follow up |
	1 + 2	3	4	5
Group A	4.8	2.6	—	3.4
Group B	5.5	3.5	2.9	4.0

Figure 7.2: Mean Prosodic Abnormality Score before and after Therapy

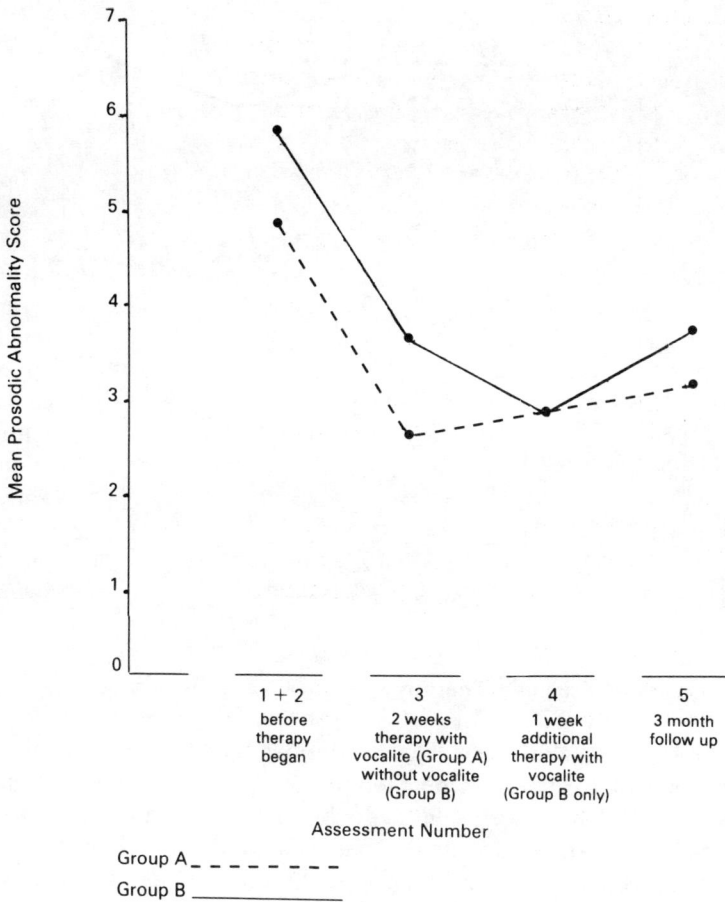

Group A _ _ _ _ _ _ _ _ _

Group B _____

Table 7.5: Effects of Therapy upon the Individual Features of Speech making up the Prosodic Abnormality Score

Feature of Speech	% of patients Affected	Improvement after Prosodic Therapy
Intonation and rhythm	100	improved marginally and maintained
Vocal quality, rate, volume	80	substantial improvement, well maintained
Pitch, tone	< 50	marginal improvement, not maintained

Figure 7.3: Assessment of Individual Features of Speech Making up the Prosodic Abnormality Score

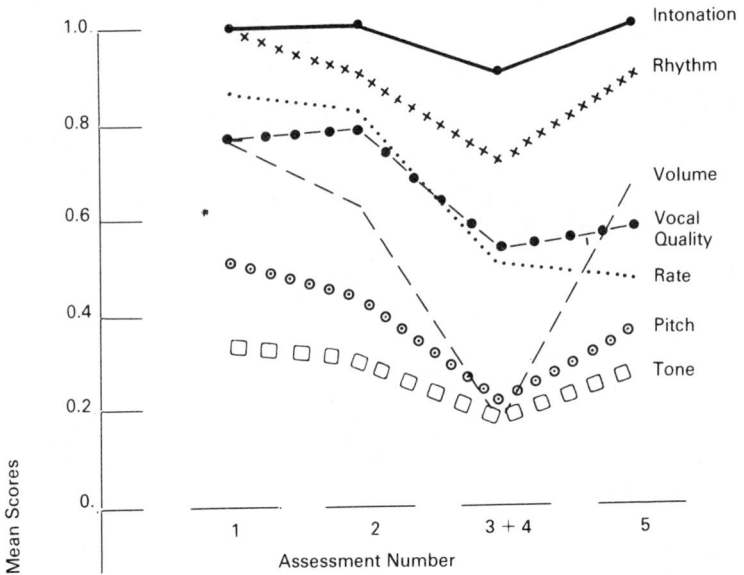

Logistics of Prosodic Therapy

Our studies make it possible to consider the logistics of a programme of treatment. One therapeutic approach is outlined in Table 7.6. There seems little doubt that the treatment should initially be carried out in the patient's own home, a common occurrence in the united Kingdom as the cost of domiciliary speech therapy may well be less than that of conveying patients by ambulance to a hospital centre. There are also substantial additional benefits in terms of contact with the patients and, even more important, with their relatives. This treatment could be envisaged during admission to hospital (but a crucial factor could be the motivation of hospital staff in maintaining any gains in communication) or on an out-patient basis in a speech therapy department or geriatric day hospital. A small trial of one week's daily group therapy, with subjects who had received daily therapy six months previously, indicated that gains lost over the six-month period could be retrieved with such intervention. It should thus be possible to use group therapy as a means of maintenance after previous intensive daily domiciliary therapy.

Group Therapy

Allan (1970) found group treatment to be of considerable benefits in Parkinson's disease. She introduced patients to articulation exercises and progressive counting to facilitate breath control, and progressed to more complex material. She emphasised that the speech improvement achieved in the clinic quickly deteriorated, and believed that unlike other dysarthric patients, who will practise daily at home, Parkinson's disease patients require constant supervision and regular review sessions, because they lack the necessary motivation; this is not our experience.

Group treatment has also been attempted on a residential holiday basis, partly financed by the Parkinson's Disease Society (see p. 57). The results of daily and individual therapy in a relaxed and friendly atmosphere proved most encouraging. An interesting feature of the holiday was the use of the hydrotherapy pool in conjunction with physiotherapy. The beneficial effects of hydrother-

Table 7 6: Recommended Ideal Therapeutic Approach

Length of treatment
Ideally this should be over a minimum of two weeks. An intensive daily regime of hourly therapy is recommended.

Place of therapy
This is best carried out on a domiciliary basis.

Therapy technique
The combined use of PNF and Prosodic Therapy, preferably using a computerised feedback device, aims to improve:
   1. Respiration — with pursed lip breathing.
   2. Swallowing — with icing exercises, taste stimulation, and tongue resistance exercises.
   3. Facial expression — muscle resistance exercises, cartoon mimicry.
   4. Intelligibility — exercises practising more normal patterns of rate, rhythm, stressing and speech emotion, intonation and vocal quality. These exercises are visually displayed on the computerised device and the patient copies them.
   5. Reception of prosody — identification and discrimination of the grammatical functions of prosody and the affective elements of speech.

apy on speech seem considerable and deserve further study (Smith, R. 1954).

The implications of such a 'vacation' approach for speech therapists may be that intensive fortnightly therapy routines occurring two or three times a year may increase the patient's motivation and encourage them to maintain their communication abilities (Robertson and Thompson, 1984). From the study by Robertson and Thompson (1984) it emerged that prior to therapy the motor speech processes are poorly integrated; following therapy these processes become more integrated into everyday communication situations. They also noted through questionnaires sent to patients and relatives that the group treatment increased their awareness and understanding of their problems; they gained in confidence and showed a desire to communicate and that they generally showed a more positive attitude to speaking. The techniques of individual and group work on motor and functional speech skills enabled the subjects to practise confidently on their own and gain increasing skill in effective functional communication.

Summary

Modern studies of methods of speech therapy intervention in Parkinson's disease indicate substantial and socially important improvements in the speech disorder of Parkinson's disease. The attitude that 'it seems impossible to discharge such patients' is changing and a more positive approach to their management emerging. Whether therapy is on an individual or group basis, a variety of proven techniques is available and in many cases, such as prosodic therapy and the 'visispeech' aids, these are not mutually exclusive but rather mutually enhancing. What is needed now is a more positive attitude from doctors for the referral of such cases to speech therapy departments.

References

Allan, C.M. (1970). Treatment of non-fluent speech resulting from neurological disease — treatment of dysarthria. *British Journal of Disorders of Communication*, 5, 1-4.

Andrews, G., and Harris, M. (1964). *The Syndrome of Stuttering.* Heinemann Medical Books, London.

Butfield, C. (1961). Dysarthria. *Speech Pathology and Therapy, 4,* 74.

Calne, D.B. (1970). *Parkinsonism: Physiology, Pharmacology and Treatment.* Edward Arnold, London.

Canter, J.G. (1963). Speech characteristics of patients with Parkinson's disease. I. Intensity pitch and duration. *Journal of Speech and Hearing Disorders, 28,* 221-9.

_____ (1965a). Speech characteristics of patients with Parkinson's disease. II. Physiological Support for Speech. *Journal of Speech and Hearing Disorders, 30,* 44-9.

_____ (1965b). Speech characteristics of patients with Parkinson's disease. III. Articulation, diadochokinesis and overall speech adequacy. *Journal of Speech and Hearing Disorders, 30,* 217-24.

Damste, P.H., and Lerman, J.W. (1975). An Introduction to Voice Pathology, Functional and Organic. C.C. Thomas, Springfield, Illinois.

Darley, F.L., Aronson, A.E., and Brown, J.R. (1975). *Motor Speech Disorders.* W.B. Saunders, Philadelphia, p. 1.

Downie, A.W., Low, J.M., and Lindsay, D.O. (1981). Speech disorder in Parkinsonism — usefulness of Delayed Auditory Feedback in selected cases. *British Journal of Disorders of Communication, 16,* 2, 135-9.

Draper, M. (1968). Aids to improving vocalisation. *New Zealand Journal of Physiotherapy, 3,* 14.

Froeschel, E. (1948). *Twentieth Century Voice Correction,* Chap. V. Philosophical Library, New York.

Greene, M.L.C. (1980). *The Voice and its Disorders.* Pitman Medical, London, pp. 298-327.

Greene, M.L.C. and Watson, B.W. (1968). The value of speech amplification in Parkinson's disease patients. *Folia Phoniatrica, 20,* 250.

Grewel, F. (1957). Classification of dysarthrias. *Acta Psychiatrica et Neurologica Scandinavica, 32,* 325-7.

Helm, N.A. (1979). Management of palilalia with a pacing board. *Journal of Speech and Hearing Disorders, 44,* 350-3.

Luria, A.R. (1967). *Traumatic Aphasia.* Mouton, The Hague.

Morley, D.E. (1955). The rehabilitation of adults with dysarthric speech. *Journal of Speech and Hearing Disorders, 20,* 58-61.

Peacher, W.G. (1947). Speech disorders in World War II. VII. Treatment of dysarthria. *Journal of Nervous and Mental Disorders, 106,* 66.

Perry, A.R. (1981). Patients with Parkinson's disease should be seen and not heard. Paper given to study day on Parkinson's disease, Glasgow.

Perry, A.R. and Das, P.K. (1981). Speech assessment of patients with Parkinson's disease. In Rose, F.C., and Capildeo, R. (eds), *Progress in Parkinson's Disease.* Pitman Medical, London, pp. 373-84.

Powers, G.L., and Starr, C.D. (1974). The effects of muscle exercises on velopharyngeal gap and nasality. *Cleft Palate Journal, 11,* 28.

Robertson, S.J. and Thomson, F. (1984). Speech therapy in Parkinson's disease. A study of the efficacy and long-term effects of intensive speech therapy. *British Journal of Disorders of Communication* (in press).

Rosenbek, J.C., and La Pointe, L.L. (1978). The dysarthrias — description, diagnosis and treatment. In Johns, D.F. (ed.), *Clinical Management of Neurogenic Communicative Disorders.* Little, Brown and Co., Boston.

Sarno, M.T. (1968). Speech impairment in Parkinson's disease. *Archives of Physical Medicine and Rehabilitation, 49,* 269.

Scott, S., and Caird, F.I. (1981). Speech therapy for patients with Parkinson's disease. *British Medical Journal, 283,* 1088.

_____ (1983). Speech therapy for Parkinson's disease. *Journal of Neurology, Neurosurgery and Psychiatry, 46,* 140-4.

_____ (1984). The response of the apparent receptive speech disorder of Parkinson's disease to speech therapy. *Journal of Neurology, Neurosurgery and Psychiatry, 47,* 302-3.

Selley, W.G. and Tudor, C. (1974). A palatal training appliance and a visual aid for use in treatment of hypernasal speech. *British Journal of Disorders of Communication, 9,* 117-22.

Smith, R.G., Bowman, I., McNiven, D.R., Scott, S. (1984). Therapeutic Holiday. Not yet published.

Smith, S. (1951). Chest register versus head register in the membrane cushion model of the vocal cords. *Folia Phoniatrica, 9,* 32-7.

Walker, S.A. (1982). Investigation into the communication effectiveness of the elderly. M. Phil Thesis, University of Leicester.

Wohl, M.T. (1968). The electronic metronome. An evaluation study. *British Journal of Disorders of Communication, 3,* 89-93.

8 ALTERNATIVE METHODS OF COMMUNICATION

The formation or retrieval of functional speech in Parkinson's disease may at times be impossible (Byers-Brown, 1981), and in such cases, alternative methods of communication require to be considered. The logic of this has not always been appreciated by those who still equate speech therapy with correction of speech. It should, however, be perfectly acceptable to a profession whose prime concern is communication, and whose ultimate goal is to develop the ability to communicate to a level adequate to meet the patient's needs. In the past clinicians have tended to regard non-speech methods as a 'last resort', introducing them only when attempts to improve speech have failed. A more positive approach to non-verbal communication as serving as an adjunct to speech as well as a substitute for it has been promoted by Silverman (1980).

Non-verbal Systems of Communication

The most commonly used non-verbal system is gesture. We all use it daily and incorporate into our personal communication system culturally determined gestures to accentuate statements. We acquire signs such as nodding of the head to indicate 'yes', and a finger to the mouth, to indicate silence; shrugging the shoulders conveys indifference or uncertainty. Our use of facial expression in particular reflects our emotional state; a smile may be a response, a signal of appeasement or a means for reducing distance. Our gaze may be welcoming or aggressive, and gaze avoidance may be used as a means for the speaker to retain the 'speaker role' (Argyle, 1969). We establish rapport through our use of bodily and facial expressions without resort to speech, and so it is easy to misunderstand the person who cannot or does not use these clues. The Parkinsonian patient is often unable to alter facial expression spontaneously, and a reduction in bodily gestures is a feature of the disease itself. Lack of facial expression and spontaneity belies the sufferer's humour and warmth of response. He may well be considered apathetic, or cold and unfeeling or even demented (Monrad-Krohn, 1956).

Many Parkinson's disease patients respond to PNF of the facial muscles (Scott and Caird, 1981). Such exercises may enable the patient to regain adequate functional movement of the face, to frown or to smile appropriately. In many instances, where the disease is in the early stages, merely drawing the patient's attention to the loss of facial expression combined with practising appropriate gestures is enough to improve their spontaneous use.

One possible method utilises facial cartoons (Figure 8.1). The use of such cartoons and a variety of materials, such as Stanley Holloway or Joyce Grenfell monologues, can provide a humorous therapy session.

Non-speech Aids

Often the patient's degree of speech handicap warrants the use of an aid. When should this choice be made? Generally a speech aid is advocated when the patient's speech is not sufficiently intelligible to convey his needs, or when speech unintelligibility (which may even be temporary) is frustrating for the patient or his relatives, or when the speech prognosis is poor despite therapeutic intervention.

Speech therapists are responsible for the diagnosis and treatment of the patient's communication problems. If assessment indicates that the prognosis for recovery of functionally adequate speech is poor, then the therapist has a responsibility to the patient to select an appropriate alternative method of communication. Ideally such an aid should be introduced gradually to the patient and not presented as a 'last resort'. The aid should be viewed as a means of relieving frustration and communication difficulty.

Many argue that aids reduce the user's motivation to speak, but Skelly (1979), studying gestural systems in dysarthric patients, found that many significantly improved their communicative abilities following the introduction of the system. Chen (1971) found similar improvements utilising a manual gesture and alphabet system.

Communication Boards

At the simplest level a communication board may be supplied.

Figure 8.1: Facial Cartoons. Instructions:
(1) Ask the patient to match the cartoon 'face' with the appropriate contextual speech clue presented by the therapist.
(2) Using a mirror, practise the selected expression from the choice of cartoons.
(3) Using contextual speech clues the patient matches his facial expression to the speech clue.
(4) Without speech clues can he alter his facial expression while the therapist or relative guesses the emotion conveyed?

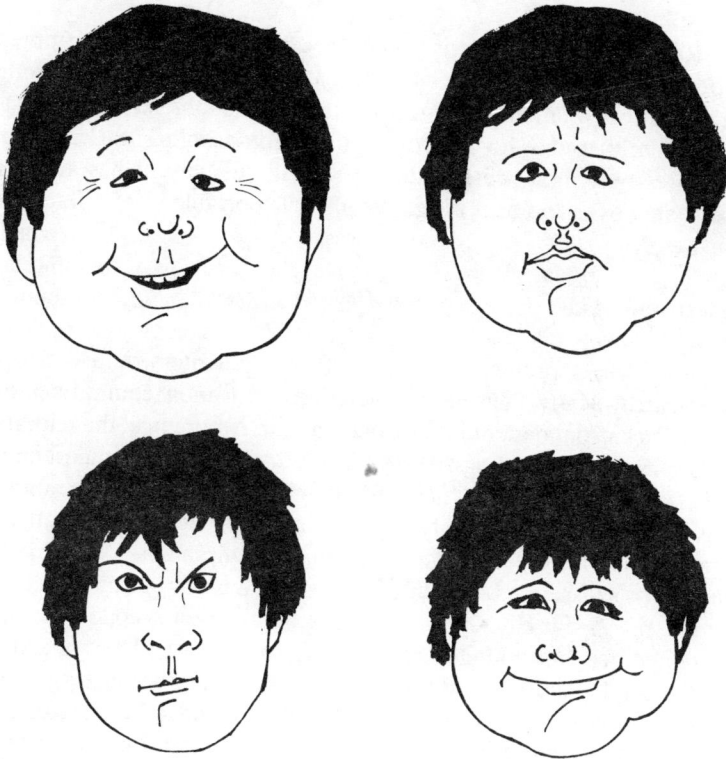

This can be adapted to suit varying degrees of manual dexterity and differing levels of complexity depending upon the individuals motor, visual and intellectual capabilities. Fawcus *et al.,* (1983) stressed that all patients with a severe communication difficulty should have access to a communication board. The only requirements are that the user is able to select or spell the message he wishes to convey and that the listener understands what is intended to be conveyed. Picture boards, such as that produced in Britain by the College of Speech Therapists, are particularly useful if the patient's comprehension is impaired. Phrase or alphabet sheets may support residual speech abilities, reinforcing or emphasising single words or phrases that the listener finds particularly difficult to understand. For efficient use these aids should be positioned in such a way that they are clearly visible to both user and listener. Often a simple table-top book-stand offers the best method of presentation. It is helpful if the board is protected with a water-resistant covering.

Recently a voice output aid (Vocaid) with pre-programmed speech has been developed. It offers a variety of overlays including alphabetical, mathematical and home-related phrase sheets. It is particularly useful for the more disabled, drooling patient, and requires only light pressure to operate the display. It has a water resistant cover and as it is lightweight it is portable.

Electronic Aids

Some patients prefer to use electronic typewriters with assisted keyboards. Many therapists have tried the Canon communicator with Parkinson patients, although in our experience the elderly find difficulty in reading and operating the keyboard. Similarly the 'tikertape' message is difficult for them to read. The Microwriter has been useful particularly with businessmen, who can adapt its many functions to suit their individual requirements. The typed facility of synthesised speech output is particularly suited to office situations. Again elderly subjects find the operation code difficult to remember, but younger subjects adapt with ease. They find the screen display a useful aid for further education or for linking with other computer modes. Similarly 'splink aids' have been adapted for these functions and like the Microwriter offer a range of print sizes for reading on paper text or screen display.

'Tools for the Living' (see Appendix 1) are willing to send information to therapists regarding the many models available.

System Selection

In order to decide upon a successful system for use many factors have to be considered, to match the needs of the user with the most appropriate aid:

(1) Ideally in progressive illness the aid should be adaptable and capable of use over a long period of time in the face of increasing disability.
(2) The patient's communication needs must be determined. The aid must be capable of providing face-to-face communication, or telephone facilities, or assistance with written communication, or the conveying of only basic needs to caring staff and relatives (or a combination of these may be the problem) and the aid appropriate to the requirements must be chosen.
(3) The patient must have adequate motor, cognitive and visual capabilities to cope with the aid and these may alter with time and the disease process.
(4) The patient must want an alternative method of communication and be motivated to use the aid if it is provided.
(5) The patient may need to use the aid himself, but will those about the patient allow him to use it? They may erroneously consider it redundant.

Summary

The use of communication aids is not 'last-resort' therapy, but active intervention. The patients rely on therapists to help them develop the appropriate attitude towards the aid. If the therapist sees it as an 'end goal' the patient can only be expected to do the same. However, a caring attitude and offering advice regarding its acceptance and best manner of use will assist the patient to overcome any embarrassment or discomfort in using the aid.

References

Argyle, M. (1969). *Social Interaction.* Tavistock Publications, London.

Byers-Brown, B. (1981). *Speech Therapy: Principles and Practice*. Churchill Livingstone, London.

Chen, L.Y. (1971). Manual communication by combined alphabet and gestures. *Archives of Physical Medicine and Rehabilitation, 52*, 381-4.

Fawcus, M., Williams, R., Williams, J., and Robinson, M. (eds) (1983). *Working with Dysphasics*. Winslow Press Ltd., Winslow, Bucks.

Monrad-Krohn, G.H. (1956). Quelques remarques sur les alterations prosodiques et leurs consequences dans la clinique neurologique. *Acta Psychiatrica et Neurologica Scandinavica, 108*, 265-7.

Scott, S., and Caird, F.I. (1981). Speech therapy for Parkinson's disease. *British Medical Journal 283*, 1088.

Silverman, F. (1980). *Communication for the Speechless*. Prentice-Hall, Englewood-Cliffs, New Jersey.

Skelly, M. (1979). *Amer-Ind Gestural Code*. Elsevier, New York.

Sonnette, C. (1982). Non-verbal communication. *Bulletin Audiophonologie, 16*, 283-92.

9 PHYSIOTHERAPY AND OCCUPATIONAL THERAPY

Patients with Parkinson's disease, certainly those in hospital, and many of those at home, will be treated by the physiotherapist and occupational therapist. Our experience is that the knowledge of speech therapists of what these other therapists aim to do in the management of Parkinsonian patients can be limited, and their need to know, at least in relevant areas, very considerable. Co-operation between therapists is essential if the patient is to derive maximum benefit from each of their activities.

Physiotherapy

In general the physiotherapist offers advice to the patient and relatives about ways of maintaining adequate trunk postures, preventing loss of mobility and improving gait.

Mobility

If a patient should experience difficulty walking into the clinic or arising from the chair at the end of the session the following may help. Place the patient in a sitting position and attempt to twist his trunk from side to side; verbal encouragement may help. Ask the patient to look as far round to the side as he can, then twist and look as far round to the other side as is possible; do this three or four times to each side. The twisting action stimulates rotation and releases the degree of immobility.

Posture

The posture adopted by the Parkinson sufferer is very important. Generally armchair support in a relaxed sitting posture is advocated. Posture can be used to facilitate increased vocal intensity — placing the patient in forearm support (Figure 9.1), i.e. when the ulnar border of the forearm is supported over a table and the patient puts his weight through it. This promotes proximal stability and fixation of the shoulder girdle and strap musculature of the neck, and increases vocal intensity.

67

Figure 9.1: The Patient's Right Hand is Supported on the Ulnar Border in the Correct Fashion — the Left is not

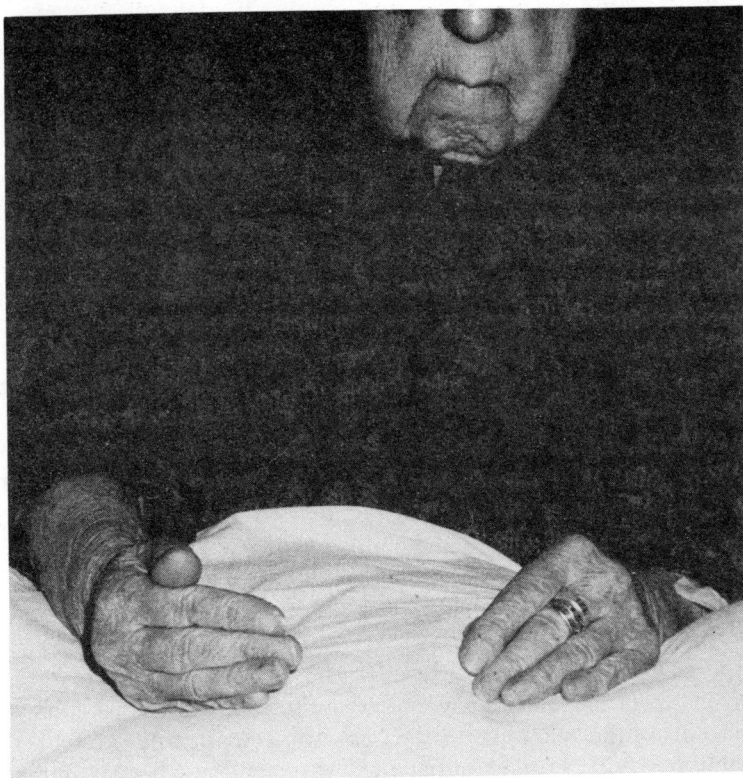

Respiration

One method which has been found to be particularly beneficial with Parkinsonian patients in facilitating diaphragmatic breathing is the pursed lip breathing technique. The patient sits in a relaxed posture with armchair support. The therapist demonstrates the technique of expiration through pursed lips, i.e. like blowing down a straw or whistling. This is followed by a pause, and then by inspiration and the repeat of expiration through pursed lips. The patient must be taught sensory awareness, i.e. the feeling of expiration. The emphasis is entirely on expiration and attention is removed from inspiration. Prior to practising the pursed lip breathing technique the patient is asked to count to ten, and the rate, volume and length of the expiratory phase are noted. Go through the sequence of steps to promote pursed lip breathing and on the final sequence as the patient is instructed to feel the air being pushed out through pursed lips, he is then instructed to count up to ten, feeling the air being pushed out during phonation. Generally there is an increase in vocal intensity and an increase in respiratory volume.

Facial Expression

Any of the upper facial movement exercises advocated by Langley and Darvill (1979) are of benefit in improving upper facial mobility. However, the muscles of the upper forehead are small and the practicalities of offering resistance to such muscles appropriately can be difficult. The exercises can be reinforced by utilising cartoons such as in Figure 8.1 and the use of phrases stressing intonational patterns. The achieving of improved facial expression can be more easily made with this multisensory bombardment. Eye hygiene, e.g. dipping cotton wool bud in ice cold water and pressing gently over the eye, pressing the eye closed and wiping the eye can often facilitate increased upper facial mobility. The physiotherapist may also improve symmetrical facial expression by tapping the cheek which stimulates facial muscles, as does stroking bilaterally near the mouth in an upward direction.

Voicing

Sucking on a small ice cube or a cube made of lemon juice can facilitate voicing in a Parkinsonian patient as can brushing to the postauricular area. *However it must be stressed that this stimulates the vagus and caution must thus be used in elderly patients who may have heart disease.* This icing, in conjunction with the pursed lip breathing, can produce immediate improvement in voicing abilities. Another method of achieving immediate voicing is to ask the patient to count to 15. When the patient stops ask him to count back from 15. Reverse counting will often bring about voicing, whereas forward counting does not.

Oral Hygiene

Many Parkinson sufferers complain of difficulty retaining dentures. The use of a thin metallic upper dental plate not only increases intra-oral tactile awareness, but it is found by many elderly patients to be easier to retain. In conjunction with the building up of the lower buccal sulcus acrylic (the acrylic of the lower denture along the gum ridge; Selley and Tudor, 1974), the increased bulk of acrylic gives the buccinator muscles a better grip and increases retention of the lower denture.

Swallowing

The exercises recommended by Langley and Darvill (1981) are recommended. Sucking on an ice cube, or icing to the lower lip will bring about tongue protrusion and possibly a swallowing reflex, particularly using an ice cube made of pure lemon juice. In conjunction with the above, exercises facilitating tongue movements resisted by a spatula will improve swallowing.

The use of taste can also bring about swallowing. A small amount of sherry dropped on closed lips from a pipette is often most effective. Cheese chewed on the back molars, lemon juice or any citrous flavour, or quinine to the back of the tongue and the velum, can produce bunching of the tongue and in conjunction with resisted tongue movement exercise will facilitate swallowing. It is important that the therapist determines the patient's taste preference prior to beginning these exercises. *It is strongly advocated that a speech therapist works in conjunction with a physiotherapist with patients who have difficulty in swallowing as therapy is potentially hazardous, i.e. the patient is prone to choking, aspiration, etc.*

Further exercises can be found in the references mentioned but the above in particular have been found most useful by the authors. Recent attempts using hydrotherapy techniques in joint physio and speech sessions during a residential holiday, were found to be most beneficial, (a) in generally relaxing the patient, (b) in improving vocalisation, and (c) in improving mobility.

Occupational Therapy

The value of the occupational therapist to the patient with Parkinson's disease is both in giving advice on the activities of daily living, and in the provision of aids which may assist these activities.

The most important areas of interest to the occupational therapist which are relevant to the speech therapist are those concerned with feeding. The most appropriate cutlery is often that with enlarged handles (Figure 9.2), which the Parkinsonian patient

Figure 9.2: Cutlery with Enlarged Handles

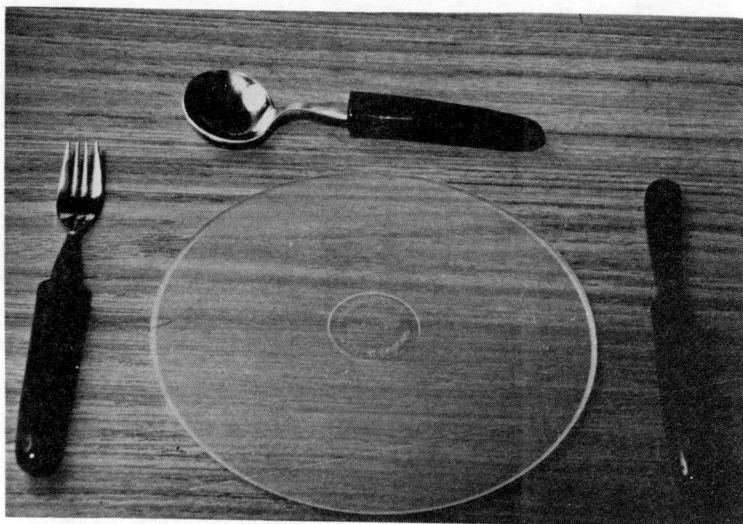

Figure 9.3: Crockery with Raised Rims to Minimise the Effects of Tremor

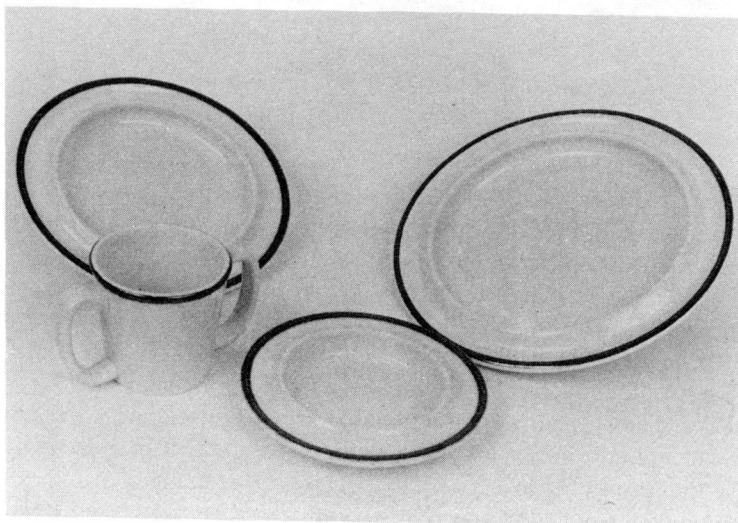

Figure 9.4: Manoy Cup and Cutlery

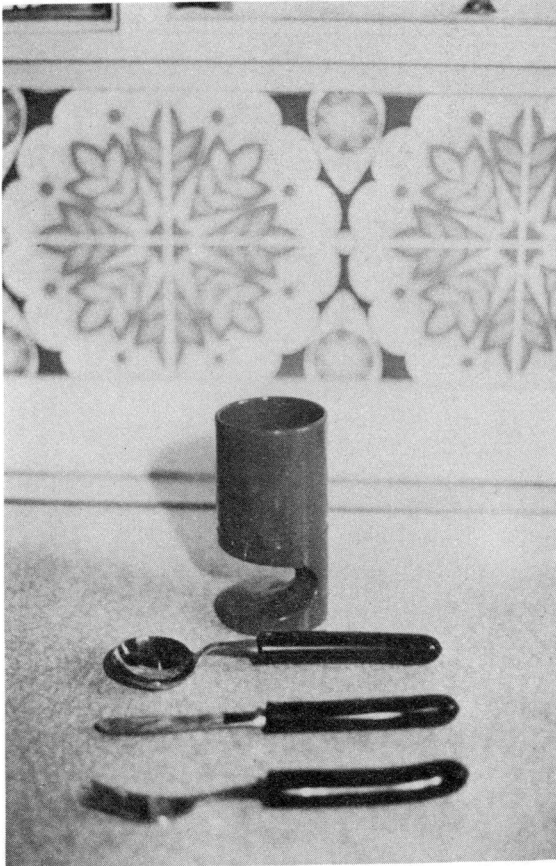

finds the easiest to manipulate accurately. Special crockery to minimise the effects of tremor in scattering food includes a variety of plates with raised rims, etc. (Figure 9.3). It is important that these should be of a type most nearly approximating those in normal use, since many of the plastic varieties cause embarrassment by their resemblance to children's plates, etc. A variety of special cups (e.g. the Manoy cup and the two-handled form) (Figure 9.4) is also available, and these may enable the Parkinsonian patient to use a cup more easily, although these too resemble babies' feeders. All the forms of crockery (and of course writing materials) are best placed on a non-slip mat (e.g. the Dycem mat, Figure 9.5), an

Figure 9.5: Dycem Non-slip Mat in Use

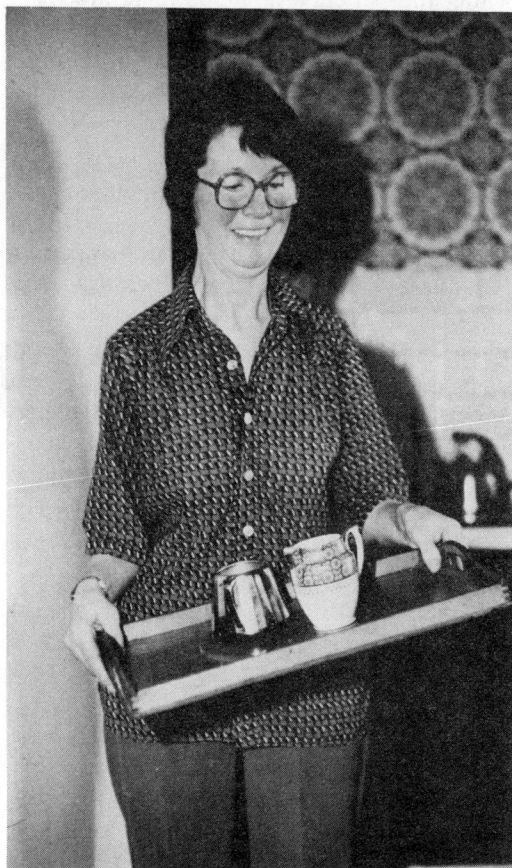

extremely simple and efficient device for preventing plates, etc., from being scattered by a tremulous hand or from slipping when a tray is inadvertently tilted.

An enlarged pencil grip and the use of Letraset will improve writing, and printing rather than script will reduce the tendency to micrographia.

All these aids may be rejected by the patient simply because they are aids, and their use marks out the patient as being disabled, but in practice most are well accepted and in fact used (Beattie and Caird, 1980). They can be provided and tested in use in the ward or day hospital, but there are as many advantages to the occupational therapist in visiting the patient's home as there are to the speech therapist. Advice can be given in a relaxed and realistic atmosphere, and rapport with and co-operation from the relatives much increased.

References

Beattie, A., and Caird, F.I. (1980). The occupational therapist and the patient with Parkinson's disease. *British Medical Journal, 163*, 1354.

Langley, J., and Darvill, G. (1979). Procedures for facilitating improvements in swallow, mastication, speech and facial expression where these have been impaired by central or peripheral nerve damage. College of Speech Therapists, London.

Selley, W.G., and Tudor, C. (1974). A palatal training appliance and a visual aid for use in treatment of hypernasal speech. *British Journal of Disorders of Communication, 9*, 117-22.

APPENDIX 1: USEFUL ADDRESSES

United Kingdom

College of Speech Therapists,
Harold Poster House,
6 Lechmere Road,
London NW2 5BU

Parkinson's Disease Society,
36 Portland Place,
London W1N 3DG

Cooper-Rand Voice Amplifiers,
Raymed (Chas Thackray Ltd.),
Viaduct Road,
Leeds, LS4 2BR

Vocalite,
Greenwood Electronics,
Unit T4,
Fullarton Road,
Tollcross,
Glasgow G32 8YL

Palatal Training Aid,
Bio Instrumentation South-West Ltd,
Holm Croft,
School Road,
Silverton,
Exeter EX5 4JH

Visual Speech Aid (Visispeech),
Royal National Institute for the Deaf,
105 Gower Street,
London WC1

Tools for the Living (Communication Aids),
P.O. Box 13,
Godalming,
Surrey GU7 1TA

USA

American Parkinson Disease Association,
116 John Street,
New York NY 10038

Parkinson's Disease Foundation,
William Black Medical Research Building,
640 West 168th Street,
New York NY 10032

United Parkinson Foundation,
220 South State Street,
Chicago,
Illinois 60604

National Parkinson Foundation,
501 N.W. 9th Avenue,
Miami,
Florida 33136

Parkinson Educational Program (PEP),
1800 Park Newport,
Suite 202-302 Newport Beach,
California 92660

Parkinsonian Foundation of Greater Washington,
3439 Fourteenth Street North,
Arlington,
Virginia 22201

Australia

Parkinson's Syndrome Society,
45 Coolaroo Road,
Lane Cove,
New South Wales 2066

Mrs E. Hemming,
Parkinson's Disease Society of Tasmania Inc.,
2 Kellatie Road,
Montagu Bay,
Hobart
Tasmania 7088

Belguim

Association pour la Lutte contre la Maladie de Parkinson, ASBL,
Vereniging Voor de Strijd Tegen de Ziekte van Parkinson VZWD,
Institut de Medecine,
Hopital de Baviere,
Bd de la Constitution 66,
4000 Liege

Canada

Parkinson's Disease Society,
1284 Clyde Avenue,
Ottawa,
Ontario K2C 1Y5

Parkinson Disease Foundation of Canada,
Manulife Centre, Suite 232,
55 Bloor Street West,
Toronto,
Ontario M4W 1A6

British Columbia Parkinson's Disease Association,
645 West Broadway,
Vancouver,
British Columbia V5Z 1G6

Denmark

Mrs Lisa Hoffmeyer,
Immortellevejo 8-2936 Vedback

Eire

Miss M.E. Macaulay,
Community & Environment Department,
Capel Buildings,
58-71 Great Strand Street,
Dublin 1

Japan

Tokyo Parkinson Patient's Association,
Abe Sueo,
3-12 Tsurumki 2-Chome,
Setagayaku,
Tokyo

Netherlands

Parkinson Patienten Vereniging Papaver,
Prinses Beatrixlaan 5,
Bunnik

New Zealand

Mrs E. Kelly,
Field Officer,
Southland Parkinson's Disease Society Inc.,
PO Box 1561,
Invercargill

Mr H.M. Schellekena,
Parkinson's Disease Society,
c/o 148 England Street,
Christchurch

N.Z. Parkinsonism Support Groups,
PO Box 11637,
Wellington

South Africa

The Secretary
South African Parkinsonian Association,
CNA Building,
39 Gale Street,
Durban
PO Box 18151,

Sweden

MS-forbundet,
Riksorganisation for neurologiskt, sjuka och handicappade,
David Bagares gata 3,
111 38 Stockholm

APPENDIX 2: PHONETIC ALPHABET

Vowels

[i] as in it
[i:] as in eat
[ɛ] as in bed
[a] as in at
[a:] as in arm
[ə:] as in her
[ə] as in supper
[ʌ] as in cut
[ɔ] as in not
[u:] as in pool

Consonants

[m] as in me
[n] as in no
[ŋ] as in sing
[p] as in pea
[b] as in bat
[t] as in to
[d] as in day
[k] as in cat
[g] as in go
[f] as in fit
[v] as in vim

[θ] as in think
[ð] as in that
[r] as in red
[j] as in yet
[s] as in so
[z] as in zoo
[ʃ] as in shoe
[tʃ] as in chat
[dʒ] as in jam
[ʒ] as in leisure
[h] as in he

Diacritics

: marking length
ı marking stress
⌃ marking pitch patterns

APPENDIX 3: DRUGS MENTIONED IN TEXT

Approved Name	Proprietary Names	
	UK	USA
amantadine	Symmetrel	Symmetrel
amitriptyline	Tryptizol	Elavil
benzhexol	Artane	Artane
(USA trihexyphenidyl)		
benztropine	Cogentin	Cogentin
bromocriptine	Parlodel	Parlodel
chlorpromazine	Largactil	Thorazine
diazepam	Valium	Valium
imipramine	Tofranil	Antipress
levodopa & benserazide	Madopar	not used
levodopa & carbidopa	Sinemet	Sinemet
lithium	Priadel	Eskalith
nitrazepam	Mogadon	Mogadon
phenytoin	Epanutin	Dilantin
prochlorperazine	Stemetil	Compazine
propranolol	Inderal	Inderal
selegiline	Eldepryl	not used
(or deprenyl)		
thioridazine	Melleril	Mellaril

APPENDIX 4: ADVICE TO RELATIVES

(1) The patient may find that to speak becomes a considerable effort. The listener must be tolerant and sympathetic towards this effort.

(2) The listener must not demand responses from the speaker that are lengthy and complex, since they will lead rapidly to fatigue. When the patient is fatigued he may have greater problems of intelligibility.

(3) Since speech intensity is reduced and its precision impaired, listeners and speakers should do whatever possible to make the environment conducive to good communication. It should be quiet and the patient should not find himself competing with extraneous noise.

(4) The speaker and listener should if possible face each other during conversation.

(5) In extreme cases of difficulty, paper and pencil, or a communication board, may allow the patient an opportunity to convey his basic needs.

(6) The listener does little to help the situation by raising his voice or exaggerating his articulatory precision. In most cases the patient's hearing and understanding are not impaired.

(7) The way in which the patient sits or stands will affect speech. He should sit with ease, be comfortable and well supported in order that he remains as relaxed as possible.

(8) Many patients find difficulty maintaining a stretch of speech. Their voices start off well, but fade away as they go on trying to talk. To overcome this, they should try to take time speaking with all sentences short and precise. It is better for them to feel they are speaking too loudly than too softly.

(9) It is important that the relatives remember that the drugs the patient takes may vary in effect throughout the day. This drug variation may also affect the speech of the sufferer; relatives should always bear this in mind.

APPENDIX 5: PREFACE TO PROSODIC FUNCTION: EXAMPLES AND EXERCISES*

Intonation is the change in pitch contour of voice sounds. It is the belief of many linguists that intonation is the first aspect of language that a child learns and, perhaps as a result of this, once learnt it is resistant to change. In English intonation permits us to convey several different messages while using the same word. Even a single word like 'yes' can indicate several different emotions depending upon how intonation is used.

Intonation and stress patterns contribute much to the meaning of entire sentences as well as individual words. Depending on how these patterns are used similar word groupings can have entirely different meanings, e.g. 'He didn't stay because I was there'. If this is spoken with slowly decreasing pitch and then a rise in pitch on the word 'I' then the presence of the speaker was not the reason the person in question stayed. However if there is a rise in pitch for the word 'didn't' this indicates that the speaker's presence was the reason why the person in question left. Obviously there are many examples of these and the following appendices offer merely some examples of their functions and phrases. It is important to mention however that the use of a visual reinforcement device to display these features can be most beneficial particularly with the more severely speech disordered patients (Scott and Caird 1981, 1983, 1984; Scott *et al.*, 1984).

The following are examples of some of the prosodic roles in speech which can be useful in therapy:

(a) Accentual Function:

> I want to gó
> I wánt to go
> Í want to go
> I want to go

(Intonation and stress locate the focus of the utterance.)

---

*The examples are of English dialect.

(b) Attitudinal Functions:
   Clipped syllables, raised pitch, fast rate may indicate anger, impatience, grim attitudes. Drawled syllables, neutral pitch, and slower rate indicate indifference. There are numerous examples.
(c) Grammatical Function: (∧denotes intonational direction, : denotes pause)
   He's ńot there! v He's not there?
(d) Listing Function:
   Would you like téa or coffee ...

   v

   Would you like tea or còffee.
(e) Elliptical Function:
   Coffee v Cóffee?
   Yours v yóurs?
(f) There are many other functions; prosodic or suprasegmental changes may alter a nominative phrase into the vocative or serve as vocal parenthesis. There are many examples and roles for consideration.

References

Scott, S., and Caird, F.I. (1981). Speech therapy for patients with Parkinson's disease. *British Medical Journal, 283*, 1088.
_____ (1983). Speech therapy for Parkinson's disease. *Journal of Neurology Neurosurgery and Psychiatry, 46*, 140-4.
_____ (1984). The response of the apparent receptive speech disorder of Parkinson's disease to speech therapy. *Journal of Neurology, Neurosurgery and Psychiatry, 47*, 302-3.
Scott, S., Caird, F.I., and Williams, B.O. (1984). Evidence for an apparent sensory speech disorder in Parkinson's disease. *Journal of Neurology, Neurosurgery and Psychiatry*, (in press).

APPENDIX 6: CONTRASTIVE STRESS DRILLS

These may be at a *phonemic* level:
    'black 'birds versus 'black birds
e.g. The crow would not consider all 'black' birds were 'black birds.
    Champagne versus sham pain
e.g. The headache from the champagne was no sham pain.

Or at a *word* level:
    Protèst (verb)   Prótest (noun)
e.g. I wish to protest about this protest.
    Recòrd (verb)   Récord (noun)
e.g. He managed to recòrd this last récord.

In therapy, examples of the above and the word drills in the following list are most useful in providing contrived patterns of stressing and intonation.

A stress drill might follow the lines of Fairbanks (1960). The clinician and the patient repeat aloud, the patient attempting to copy the therapist's model of intonation and stressing.

e.g.	Clinician:	1.	Bob bit Bill
	Clinician:		Did Bob bite Bill?
	Patient:		Yes! Bob bit Bill
	Clinician:		Did Bill bite Bob?
	Patient:		No! Bob bit Bill
	Clinician:		Who bit Bill?
	Patient:		Bob bit Bill

Word Lists:

Presented for individual practice then as contrastive pairs they act as an amusing, if somewhat contrived mode, to slow rate and improve stressing.

Farthing		Banner Centre
Far thing	Ban her	Sent her
Compete	Double	Four candles
Come Pete	Dub Bill	Fork handles
Why choose	Waiter	Packet
White shoes	Wait here	Pack it
Bank here	Peace talks	Lender
Banker	Pea stalks	Lend her
Candle	Counted	Carpet
Can deal	Count Ted	Car pet
I scream	Handed	Single
Ice cream	Hand dead	Sing Gail
Tanker	Nitrate	Fankled
Tank her	Night rate	Fan Killed
Canny	House trained	Daughter
Can he	How strained	Doubt her
Willie	A name	Ticket
Will he	An aim	Tick it

Paired sentences may then be presented for completion:
  e.g. Complete the following with the correct phrase:

1. She had broken her arm so the ...
    This is the proper ...
  Answer:
      Way to cut it
      Waiter cut it

2. He was ...
    Oh! good you can ...
  Answer:
      Counted in
      Count Ted in

Rhythm and Rate:

(1) Utilising natural speech rhythms facilitates more normal prosodic patterning and rate. For example, the saying aloud of:
multiplication tables
limericks
football results
or popular verses or odes such as those by Pam Ayres and Cyril
Fletcher.
These are usually short and most obviously lyrical.
(2) Syllabic sequencing may be useful in overcoming initiation difficulties:

e.g.	big	bigger	biggest
	man	manner	manifold
	my	mine	miner
	sum	summer	something

Reference

Fairbanks, G. (1960). *Voice and Articulation Drill Book*, 2nd edn.
Harper & Row, New York.

APPENDIX 7: PROSODIC ABNORMALITY ASSESSMENT (UNIVERSITY OF GLASGOW, DEPARTMENT OF GERIATRIC MEDICINE, ASSESSMENT OF THE SPEECH DISORDER OF PARKINSON'S DISEASE)

TRIAL NO: ASSESSMENT DATE:

TAPE NO:

NAME: SEX: AGE:

REFERRAL SOURCE:

ONSET:

HEARING ACUITY:

VISUAL ACUITY:

PHYSICAL DEFICIT:

HANDEDNESS:

INTELLECTUAL LEVEL: OCCUPATION:

SWALLOWING:

CONCOMITANT ILLNESS:

DRUG REGIME:

PREVIOUS MEDICAL HISTORY:

PREVIOUS FAMILY HISTORY:

Scoring System: Prosodic Analysis

Normal scores nought. Any abnormality scores 1. Individual features score qualitatively only. *Articulation test scoring*: scores 1 for each error made.

Scoring Profile	Normal	Score	Max. Error
Feature Assessed			
1. Prosodic abnormality	0		7
2. Respiratory function	0		6
3. Phonatory function	0		6
4. Articulatory agility	0		18
5. Articulation test	0		128

Parkinson Assessment

Trial No:
Tape No.

			Test 1	2	3	4
A.	VOLUME	Loud				
		Mono				
		Normal				
		Quiet				
		Fading				
		Improved				
B.	PITCH	High				
		Low				
		Normal				
		Monotone				
		Breaks				
C.	TONE	Hyper				
		Mixed				
		Normal				
		Hypo				
D.	INTONATION	Monotone				
		Reduced				
		Normal				
		Inappropriate				
		Improved				
E.	VOCAL QUALITY	Hoarse				
		Strident				
		Normal				
		Tremor				
		Aphonic				
F.	RATE	Too fast				
		Progressively increasing in speed				
		Normal				
		Progressively decreasing in speed				
		Slow				
		Improved				
G.	RHYTHM	Stammerlike				
		Insufficient stressing				
		Normal				
		Inappropriate silences				
		Improved				
		PROSODIC ABNORMALITY SCORE				
	INTELLIGIBILITY	Normal				
		Understandable if listened carefully				
		Single words understandable but difficult to follow				
		Unintelligible				
TOTAL PROSODIC ABNORMALITY SCORE						

A. *Respiration*

Description	At Rest		For Speech		Comment
Diaphragmatic	Present	Absent	Present	Absent	
Regular					
Synchronised with Phonation					
Clavicular					
Rapid					
Slow					
Irregular					
Speaks on Residual Air					
Speaks on Ingressive Air-stream					
Comments					
Range: 0-6 Score:					

B. Phonation

	Present	Absent	Comment
Initiation Loudness Appropriate Loudness Variation Able to Repeat Voicing (A; A; A) Phonation Time (9 secs average normal)			
Voice Quality Normal (Modal)			
Harsh/Rough Creak Strident Spasticity Phonatory Loss (ES) Breathy Tension Tremulous Voice Stoppages (Associated Glottal Closure)			
Range: 0-6 Score:			

C. *Articulatory Agility*

	At Rest	For Speech	Range	Rate	Comment
Lips Symmetry					
Rounding					
Pursing					
Stretching					
Alternating movements					
Tongue Symmetry					
Protrusion					
Retraction					
Lat. movements					
Elevation					
Depressing					
Grooving					
Tremor					
Fasciculation					
Palate Symmetry					
Functional in speech					
Facial Musculature Symmetry Wasting					
Range: 0-18 Score:					

Articulation Testing

Score 1 for each correct sound

PIE
BOY
TEA
DO
CAR
GO
FOUR
VAN
THIGH
THAT
SEA
ZOO
SHY
BEIGE
CHAIR
JOY
LIE
RAN
WHY
HIGH
MY
YOU
NO
SING
WAY

Consonant Position

Ability to read sentences and/or repeat sounds. Score 1 for each correct sound.

PICK THE RIPE APPLES
A TUBE OF BABY CREAM
PUT OUT THE BUTTER FOR TEA
THE GARDEN IS HARD TO DIG
THE CAT IS DRINKING MILK
THE DOG IS IN THE GARDEN AGAIN

HE TELEPHONED FOR A GAME OF GOLF
DRIVE THE VAN TO THE RIVER
THANKS FOR BOTH BIRTHDAY CARDS
BATHE THE BOY'S BROTHER
SALLY WENT MISSING AT THE POLICE STATION
THE ZOO HAS A CHIMPANZEE MAZE
SHE WASHED A BRUSH
BEIGE AND AZURE ARE COLOURS
YOUR WATCH IS ON THE KITCHEN CHAIR
THE BADGER JUMPED OFF THE BRIDGE
ALL THE LEAVES HAVE FALLEN
A RED CHERRY CAR
THROW THE WATER AWAY
HE WAS AHEAD OF HER
YOU FETCH THE MAYOR
THE CAMERA IS IN MY ROOM
THE MAN HAD NO MONEY
THAT SINGER! BRING HER TO ME
A WHILE AGO IT WAS WHITE

Polysyllabic Words

ENCYCLOPAEDIA
AUTOBIOGRAPHY
MISSISSIPI
ASSASSINATION
HYPOCRITICAL
SECRETARY
SUBTLETY
KALEIDOSCOPE
IDIOSYNCRASY
PERMANENCY
ILLUSTRIOUS
ALTRUISTIC

Reading Passages

FROM SCARBOROUGH TO WHITBY IS A VERY PLEA-
SANT JOURNEY, WITH VERY BEAUTIFUL COUNTRY-
SIDE. IN FACT THE YORKSHIRE COAST IS LOVELY,

ALL ALONG, EXCEPT THE PARTS THAT ARE
COVERED IN CARAVANS OF COURSE, AND IF YOU GO
IN SPRING, WHEN THE GORSE IS OUT, OR IN SUMMER,
WHEN THE HEATHER'S OUT, IT IS REALLY ONE OF
THE MOST DELIGHTFUL AREAS IN THE WHOLE
COUNTRY.

THE MOORLAND IS RATHER HIGH UP, AND FAIRLY
FLAT — A SORT OF PLATEAU. AT LEAST, IT ISN'T FLAT,
WHEN YOU GET UP ON TOP; IT'S ROLLING MOOR-
LAND CUT ACROSS BY STEEP VALLEYS. BUT SEEN
FROM THE COAST IT'S UP THERE ON THE MOORS;
AND YOU ALWAYS THINK OF IT AS A KIND OF TABLE
LAND.

THE HEATHER GROWS RIGHT TO THE EDGE OF THE
HIGH GROUND, AND WHERE THIS ENDS THERE'S A
STEEP SLOPE WITH WOODS AND FIELDS. THEN
THERE'S A CERTAIN AMOUNT OF FARMLAND,
WHERE THE GROUND LEVELS OUT A BIT, WITH
CROPS AND PASTURE — AND FINALLY YOU COME TO
THE CLIFFS, THE CLIFFS THAT RUN ALONG THE
SHORE, SLOPING DOWN TO THE SEA. THESE CLIFFS
ARE VERY HIGH IN SOME PLACES, AND VERY SHEER,
AND THEY TEND TO CRUMBLE AND FALL INTO THE
SEA. ONE OF THE THINGS YOU HAD TO BE CAREFUL
ABOUT WAS NOT TO WALK TOO NEAR THE EDGE OF
THE CLIFF, BECAUSE IT'S FULL OF RABBIT HOLES,
AND IF YOU DO WALK TOO NEAR THE EDGE THE
WHOLE CLIFF'S LIABLE TO FALL AWAY UNDER-
NEATH YOU.

APPENDIX 8: COMPILATION OF EXERCISES FOR PROSODIC THERAPY

These exercises are based on M.A.K. Halliday, *A Course in Spoken English: Intonation* (Oxford University Press, 1970). Clarity of speech is dependent upon short phrasing. Note:

(1) Take time to consider what you wish to say.
(2) Think about breathing.
(3) Keep all sentences short; *do not* carry on talking when breath has run out.
(4) Try and think about making each phrase you say sound terribly interesting.
(5) *Use* your face to convey meaning.

Ideally therapy should commence as soon as possible, but length of illness or severity of illness need not exclude patients from active and effective intervention. The following exercises were used on a daily domiciliary basis over a two/three week period with good results (see Chapter 7). Each session lasted 40 minutes to one hour and there was a good degree of carry-over when therapy stopped at the end of three weeks, many patients maintaining progress for up to three months. The exercises have also been used successfully on a group basis.

The removal of emphasis from articulatory clarity and precision to more normal patterns of conversational speech appeared to maintain the patient's interest and was self-reinforcing. The exercises may be used alone or in conjunction with the Vocalite or Visispeech aids. Some punctuation is omitted to allow the therapist or patient to convey individual and varying interpretations of the phrases.

When reading aloud the therapist stresses the underlined segments and the patient copies. Initially the words and phrases may be said as statements. Then varying intonations may be introduced. The patient reads the practised phrases aloud to the therapist who copies the performance, requesting if stressing, intonation, etc. are correct. For the rhythm phrases on page 87, each section has a similar stressing rhythm. The patient and therapist tap out the rhythm and then the patient tries to fit the phrases into the correct pattern. In the set of exercises following these, the bracketed instructions predetermine the context of the phrase. After reading the bracketed part silently, the patient says aloud the phrase, implying what was written in the bracket. Then, finally, note that the reading passages and articulatory agility exercises are *not* for speed of utterance but rather to achieve controlled, deliberate production.

All the exercises have been used with very severe patients. The time taken over each section varies according to the patient's ability. The list is not a final one. Each section is left open-ended for the therapist or patient to add to or amend, and merely serves as an example.

Procedure:
    (1) Read aloud, emphasising underlined portion.
    (2) Concentrate on clarity and phrasing.

A.   Yours
       Gone
       First
       Sugar
       <u>Te</u>lephone
       All visitors a<u>shore</u>
       <u>Li</u>verpool Street.
       How can you <u>say</u> that
       <u>Hir</u>ing wouldn't cost you very much
       <u>Jane's</u> looking pleased with herself.
       <u>Ei</u>leen
       Pretty as a <u>pic</u>ture
       <u>Fin</u>ally
       Don't you want to go <u>first</u> for a change
       So
       <u>Phone</u> them and <u>ask</u> them.
       <u>Robert</u> never does any <u>gardening</u>.
       <u>Seems</u> like it
       Don't be so <u>sure</u> of yourself
       <u>Pi</u>ano sonata.
       <u>When</u> did you say, you'd able able to give me the <u>money</u>, I
         lent you

All change
<u>No</u> one would like it.
<u>por</u>ter madam,
<u>Could</u>n't they
Goal
<u>Wait</u>ing doesn't bother me.
George
<u>Hon</u>estly
Shakespeare exhibition
<u>Isn't there enough</u>
<u>Mar</u>vellous
<u>Rub</u>bish
Great
Catch
Look
Choose
<u>Train</u>s were late, <u>buses</u> were late.
<u>New</u>castle
Wasn't it a <u>strange story</u> he was telling.

B. Is that cheese to <u>eat</u> or is it to put in a <u>mouse</u> trap?
    If I'd known <u>earli</u>er about the wedding I'd have sent a <u>cable</u>.
    You're waiting to see the <u>surgeon</u>, <u>are</u> you?
    What's the <u>hurry</u>? Why not stay and <u>talk</u> for a while?
    I can leave it on the <u>table</u> and you can get it whenever you
        <u>want</u> it.
    They haven't any proper <u>control</u> over all these <u>building</u>
        schemes.
    I'll promise anything you <u>like</u> if only you'll take that <u>hat</u> off.
    It's only force of <u>habit</u>; I'm quite <u>happy</u> to change.
    She was ninety-<u>eight</u> when she <u>died</u>.
    We never disa<u>gree</u>, <u>do</u> we? Oh <u>no</u>!
    We saw some <u>marvellous</u> things in <u>Moscow</u>.
    As soon as I get to the <u>office</u> the <u>telephone</u> starts <u>ringing</u>.
    Put it <u>back</u> if you don't <u>want</u> it.
    He's done some very interesting <u>research</u> in the field of
        <u>animal</u> be<u>haviour</u>, there's just a chance he might get a
        <u>scholarship</u> if he <u>really</u> works <u>hard</u>.
    Have you seen the <u>silks</u> we got from <u>France</u>?
    There's time and a place for <u>everything</u>.
    It wasn't <u>my</u> fault.

What's the <u>matter</u>, are they all <u>dumb</u>?
Is that the <u>Cast</u>le up there, or is it a disused <u>rail</u>way station?
I haven't the slightest <u>inten</u>tion of putting <u>Rob</u>ert in charge.
<u>Stone</u> would look better than <u>brick.</u>
I don't think he looks very <u>well</u>, do <u>you</u>?
That <u>can't</u> be <u>them</u> yet, <u>can</u> it?
That's our new <u>manager</u>, the one that's just been ap<u>pointed</u>.
They don't get any more than their <u>share</u>.
If they don't pull down that old mill chimney <u>soon</u> it'll <u>fall</u>
   down.
Have you any old ma<u>gazine</u>s you wouldn't mind giving
away?
It's not a very <u>easy</u> piece of music to listen to, but I en<u>joyed</u>
   it.
On the Isle of <u>Man</u> you can still ride in a horse-drawn <u>tram</u>.
I was lying on the <u>grass</u> dreaming of all the people I'd
   <u>known</u> here.
Could Mr <u>Twenty</u>man come to the <u>tele</u>phone please?
Guess who's <u>here</u>?
That house on the <u>green</u> is probably early <u>Geor</u>gian, isn't it?
Climbing that North Face in this <u>weather</u>, <u>I ask</u> you!
There's a beautiful pattern of <u>ice</u> formed on that <u>wind</u>ow.
A couple of pints of beer a <u>day</u> and that's about the <u>lot</u>!
I'll <u>answer</u> it,
It cost one and elevenpence <u>half</u>penny.
Would you say there are <u>fewer</u> cases of snake bite <u>now</u> than
   there used to be, doctor, or <u>more</u>?

Now read the following aloud. Concentrate on the rhythm of the phrase.

A.   I think so
     glottal stop
     Can't be done
     That's a lie
     Sounds great
     Cottage chese
     Chrysanthemum
     Bachelor pad
     Photo gravure
     She came with us

At breakfast
Not enough
Turnip souffle

B.   Lentil vinagrette
I didn't know the way
Put it on the shelf
Waiting for the train
Some half-eaten buns
Frankfurt for connections
Interrogate them
Empiricism
I wanted you to know
It's quicker by bus
They wanted us to
Saffron rice with peas
Rattle-wielding fans
You need a haircut

C.   When can I speak to the boss?
Permissive society
I'd like a glass of beer
A slight attack of jaundice
They've left Yugoslavia
Alistair went to the game
A glass of beer is what I need
A gallon of paraffin
On Friday afternoon
The concert starts at eight
Impenetrability
He left the room without a word.
You can tell a man that boozes.

D.   I wanted you to write about it.
You'd best be as quick as you can.
The train is more convenient than the bus.
A spoonful of apricot jam
The ambulance took him to hospital
I'd like it with some soda water
An apple a day keeps the doctor away
I didn't expect to be asked

In the following rhythm phrase exercise:
   (1) Read aloud and emphasise the syllable underlined.
   (2) Try to make sense of the phrase
      (a) Is it a question?
      (b) Is it a statement?
      Use your voice appropriately to convey the differences.

Seven fives are thirty <u>five</u>
I wonder if there's any <u>left</u>
Leave it a-<u>lone</u>
Peter wants us to go for a <u>ride</u> in his new <u>car</u>
It's the third turning on the <u>right</u>
One pound three and <u>nine</u>
Where can I leave my <u>coat</u>
I don't know how much he <u>wants</u>
Why did you lead a spade
Let's go and see if we can get a copy of the <u>report</u>
They couldn't have done it any more <u>cheaply</u>
Single to <u>Exeter</u>
I'll meet you outside the <u>Cinema</u>
It's entirely un-<u>necessary</u>
Ladies and <u>gentlemen</u>
Where did you put my German <u>dictionary</u>.
The twenty <u>fifth</u> of April
Nineteen <u>seventy</u>.
Throw it out of the <u>window</u>
He lost his seat in one of the mid-term <u>by</u>-elections.
Who told <u>Granny</u>.
I think it's rather too <u>fancy</u>, don't <u>you</u>?
How much are iced <u>lollies</u> please?
He <u>loves</u> to spend his weekends in the <u>garden</u>
On the <u>face</u> of it, what he says, is quite <u>valid</u>
They don't even do their <u>own</u> job properly!
You ought to go and see the <u>doctor</u> if it doesn't get <u>better</u>
Did you get any <u>walking</u> or <u>climbing</u>?
Is it half past <u>eleven</u> already?
One false <u>move</u> and you're ruined for <u>life</u>
Give my regards to <u>Arthur</u>
Not many people <u>know</u> about the place <u>actually</u>
Are you <u>sure</u> they were going to come and meet you?
You think it's rather too <u>fancy</u> do you?

Sing us a <u>song</u> and we'll all join in the <u>chorus</u>
You never take <u>advice</u> from anyone, <u>do</u> you?
When <u>I</u> was young there wasn't all this hooliganism
They might even suspect <u>you</u> if you don't shave off that <u>beard</u>
    of yours.
The <u>manager</u>'s waiting to see you
Doesn't <u>Bill</u> live here any more?
Do you really <u>think</u> it suits me or were you just being <u>kind</u>?
It's absolutely no use trying to convince him he's <u>wrong</u>.
<u>Yes</u> please!
<u>Hundr</u>eds of people were arrested
I pre<u>sume</u> so
If you turn it <u>over</u> you can see what's written on the <u>back</u> of
    the paper
There's no time to <u>lose</u>
Your <u>turn</u>
What a complete waste of <u>time</u> that was
Haven't you ever <u>been</u> to the Tower of London?
Is Robert <u>coming</u> then or <u>isn't</u> he?
Isn't there a <u>post</u> office here or a <u>telegraph</u> office or some-
    thing.
<u>Idiot</u>!
They ought to be building schools and <u>hospitals</u> rather than
    blocks of <u>offices</u>
Approximately
<u>Summ</u>er they call it
<u>Silk</u> doesn't crush
The more you <u>hurry</u> them the slower they <u>get</u>.
I <u>told</u> you it <u>might</u> <u>bite</u> you
But <u>all</u> my family have curly hair
There's no harm in <u>asking</u> for it.

Now in the following read the part in brackets — to yourself. This
determines the meaning of the sentence. Having determined the
meaning:

  (1) Read the phrase aloud. Concentrate on emphasis and
  intonation to convey the meaning required.
  (2) Some phrases may require the rate to be slower for effect.
  Take time.
  (3) When listing, each unit requires some degree of emphasis
  but the last unit requires more to denote completion.

(4) For the last two pairs, the patient or therapist may use their own selection of situational clue.

red white and blue (... are my favourite colours)
red white and blue (... is my favourite colour combination)

bacon and eggs (... that's what we need from the shop)
bacon and eggs (... for breakfast)

Philip, and George, are getting married (both of them)
Philip and Jean are getting married (to each other)

they walked backwards and forwards (did they walk backwards?)
they walked backwards and forwards (in both directions)

knife fork and spoon (all three)
knife fork and spoon (the set)

is it Daphne's?
is it Daphne's (surely not?)

are we on time? (we should be)
are we on time? (are we early? we shouldn't be)

have you lost it? (never mind!)
have you lost it? (oh dear!)

all by her self (good!)
all by her self (I don't believe it)

have you got a dictionary? (as a matter of interest)
have you got a dictionary? (that's what I need!)

careful
careful?

look out (watch it, it'll sting you)
look out (watch it, I warned you)

Michael, you'd better hurry (they're expecting you)
Michael, you'd better hurry (I'm getting impatient)

never mind (it's not your business)
never mind (don't worry; it doesn't matter)

good morning (salutation)
good morning (angrily)

good night (angry valediction)
good night (normal)

I know (you needn't tell me)
I know (I understand)

after you (you should go first)
after you (normal politeness)

he's quite tame (don't worry!)
he's quite tame (don't fuss! What's all the fuss about?)

you needn't hurry (reassuring)
they needn't hurry (casual)

no-one will notice
no-one will notice

You must meet my cousin the bank manager (defining: e.g. I have
    more than one cousin, or his being a bank manager is the reason
    for meeting him)
You must meet my cousin the bank manager (non-defining: e.g. I
    have only one cousin, or his being a bank manager is incidental)

He's standing by the tree with a hat on (the tree has a hat on)
He's standing by the tree with a hat on (he has a hat on)

She sings and dances too (in addition to acting, she sings and
    dances)
She sings and dances too (in addition to singing, she dances)
She sings and dances too (amazement)

it's me Alison (Alison! it's me!)
it's me Alison (I'm Alison)

it's all taken care of
it's all taken care of

it's for their own good
it's for their own good

Now, for the next exercise read the part in brackets to yourself. This determines the meaning of the sentence. Read it first, think about the meaning it conveys and say the phrase in an appropriate form — matching the situational clue.

He speaks French, English, German and Russian
Two and six, five, seven and six, ten (your change, madam!)
Animal, vegetable and mineral
Twenty seven, twenty eight, twenty nine, thirty, thirty one, thirty two.
You can have chicken or veal or beef or liver.
Monday, Tuesday, Wednesday, Thursday, Friday, Saturday
A grapefruit, two oranges, a pount of apples, and a lemon.
Cuxton, Halling, Snodlands, Newhithe, Aylesford, Maidstone Barracks and Maidstone West (Change at Strood for ...)
The ace of hearts, the king and queen of spades, and two small diamonds.
Sun, moon and stars
Would you like to see the presents I got?
Can I see what Andrew gave you
(I'm sure he would give you something nice)
Would a nail file do (have you got a screwdriver?)
Is that the managing director (... that insignificant fellow there?)
Where's the clothesbrush (... please? I need it)
Does every one here run a Rolls Royce (... are they all so rich?)
D'you think we can get some coffee in this miserable place (I'd like some, but it seems rather unlikely)
Couldn't you see he was coming straight towards you (... I thought it was obvious)
Haven't you got a stronger bulb than this (... this one's hardly bright enough to read by!)

Reading Passages

1. From Scarborough to <u>Whitby</u> is a very pleasant <u>journey</u>, with very beautiful <u>countryside</u>. In fact the Yorkshire coast is <u>lovely</u>, all along, <u>except</u> the parts that are covered in <u>caravans</u> of course, and if you go in <u>spring</u>, when the <u>gorse</u> is out, or in <u>summer</u>, when the <u>heather's</u> out, it is really one of the most <u>delightful areas</u> in the whole <u>country</u>.

    The <u>moorland</u> is rather high <u>up</u>, and fairly <u>flat</u> — a sort of <u>plateau</u>. At <u>least</u>, it <u>isn't flat</u>, when you get up on <u>top</u>; it's rolling <u>moorland</u> cut across by steep <u>valleys</u>. But seen from the <u>coast</u> it's up there on the <u>moors</u>; and you always <u>think</u> of it as a kind of <u>table</u> land.

    The heather grows right to the <u>edge</u> of the high <u>ground</u>, and where this <u>ends</u> there's a steep <u>slope</u> with <u>woods</u> and <u>fields</u>. Then there's a certain amount of <u>farmland</u>, where the ground levels <u>out</u> a bit, with <u>crops</u> and <u>pasture</u> — and finally you come to the <u>cliffs</u>, the cliffs that run along the <u>shore</u>, sloping down to the <u>sea</u>. These <u>cliffs</u> are very <u>high</u> in <u>some</u> places, and very <u>sheer</u>, and they tend to <u>crumble</u> and fall into the <u>sea</u>. One of the things you had to be <u>careful</u> about was not to walk too near the <u>edge</u> of the cliff, because it's full of <u>rabbit</u> holes, and if you <u>do</u> walk too near the edge the whole <u>cliff's</u> liable to fall away under<u>neath</u> you.

2. The <u>beach</u> is <u>fascinating</u> like <u>all</u> beaches. There's quite an expanse of <u>sand</u>; but also lots of little spurs of <u>rock</u> jutting out into the <u>sea</u>, and <u>these</u>, of <u>course</u>, are covered in tiny <u>pools</u> with all sorts of interesting marine <u>life</u> in them: crabs and limpets and mussels and sea anemones and I don't know <u>what</u>. And sometimes you can pick up semi precious <u>stones</u> among the <u>pebbles</u>: Cor<u>ne</u>lian and <u>A</u>gate and such like.

    It's a <u>wonderful</u> place to be able to roam and wander where you <u>like.</u> One of the <u>greatest</u> pleasures I can remember was finding little <u>streams</u> that ran down the moors into the <u>sea</u>. You start at the <u>mouth</u> of the stream and you follow it up to its <u>source</u>, up on the <u>moors</u>, where it <u>starts</u> its life as no more than a boggy patch of ground. Come to think of it, I don't know any better pastime for spending a carefree summer's day.

Exercises for Agility and Phrasing

Procedure:

(a) Read quietly to familiarise subject with material.
(b) Read aloud very slowly but meaningfully.
(c) Try to build up speed but maintain clarity.

(1)   I snuff shop snuff, do you snuff shop snuff?
(2)   Should such a shapely sash such shabby stitches show?
(3)   She sells sea shells, sherry, and sand-shoes.
(4)   And ere her ear had heard, her heart had heard.
(5)   The suitability of a suet pudding without superfluous plums, is a superstition presumably due to Susan's true economy.
(6)   He generally reads regularly in a government library particularly rich in Coptic manuscripts except during the month of February.
(7)   This lute, with its flute-like tones, was captured in the loot of a great city, and its luminous sides, are made of unpolluted silver.
(8)   She sees a shot-silk sash-shop, full of Surak silk sashes, where the sun shines on the shop signs.
(9)   She is a thistle sifter, and she has a sieve of sifted thistles, and a sieve of unsifted thistles, because she is a thistle sifter.
(10)   The Duke, paid the money due to the Jew, before the dew was off the grass on Tuesday, and the Jew, having duly acknowledged it, said adieu, to the Duke, for ever.

GLOSSARY

Blepharoclonus: Rhythmical contractions of the musculature of the eyelids.

Blepharospasm: Spasm of the eyelids.

Cataract: Partial or complete opacity of the lens of the eye.

Diadochokinesia: The ability to make rapid alternating movements.

Dysarthria: Speech disorder of neurological origin.

Dysarthrophonia: Neuromuscularly-based disorder of speech affecting phonation and articulation.

Dyskinesia: Abnormal involuntary movements.

Dysphasia: The inability to interpret or formulate words manifested in listening, reading, speaking, gesture and writing.

Dysphonia: Impairment of voice.

Electrolaryngograph: Electrical device for registering the laryngeal movements.

Encephalitis: Inflammation of the brain.

Glaucoma: Eye disease characterised by raised intra-ocular pressure.

Oculogyric crises: Spasmodic conjugate deviations of the eye.

Orthostatic hypotension: Abnormally low blood pressure on assuming an erect posture.

Ossification: The process of bone formation.

Pathognomonic: Characteristic, or indicative of, a given disease.

Plastic: 'Lead-pipe' rigidity of the musculature.

Phoneme: The minimal functionally contrastive unit of sound.

Phonological: Pertaining to the study of the sound system of a language.

Presbyacusis: The deterioration of hearing with advancing age.

Prosody: All vaiations of time, pitch and loudness that accomplish emphasis, interest or individual modes of expression in speech.

Sebum: The secretions of the sebaceous glands.

Suprasegmental: Speech signals denoting emotional states.

Velum: Soft-palate.

Xeroradiography: Dry photo-electric process for recording X-ray images.

INDEX

Ideas about music & speech in (?)

Hearing effect –

eg: read words of well-known song
a) sing it | b) repeat it
read again ?? any improvement